IUPAB Biophysics Series
sponsored by
The International Union of Pure and Applied Biophysics

Photoreceptors

Their role in vision

IUPAB Biophysics Series

sponsored by

The International Union of Pure and Applied Biophysics

Editors:

Franklin Hutchinson
Yale University

Watson Fuller
University of Keele

Lorin J. Mullins
University of Maryland

Raimundo Villegas
IVIC, Caracas

1 Walter Harm: Biological effects of ultraviolet radiation
2 Stanley G. Schultz: Basic principles of membrane transport
3 Edward G. Richards: An introduction to the physical properties of large molecules in solution
4 Roderick K. Clayton: Photosynthesis: physical mechanisms and chemical patterns
5 Alan Fein and Ete Z. Szuts: Photoreceptors: their role in vision

Photoreceptors
Their role in vision

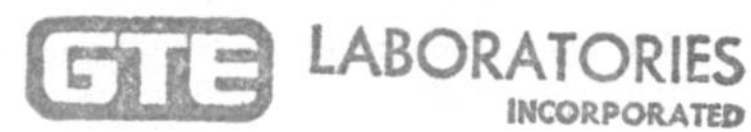

ALAN FEIN and ETE Z. SZUTS

Marine Biological Laboratory
Woods Hole, Massachusetts

CAMBRIDGE UNIVERSITY PRESS
CAMBRIDGE
LONDON NEW YORK NEW ROCHELLE
MELBOURNE SYDNEY

Published by the Press Syndicate of the University of Cambridge
The Pitt Building, Trumpington Street, Cambridge CB2 1RP
32 East 57th Street, New York, NY 10022, USA
296 Beaconsfield Parade, Middle Park, Melbourne 3206, Australia

First published 1982

Printed in the United States of America

Library of Congress Cataloging in Publication Data

Fein, Alan, 1942–

Photoreceptors, their role in vision.

(IUPAB biophysics series; 5)

Includes bibliographical references and index.

1. Photoreceptors. 2. Vision. I. Szuts, Ete Z. (Zoltan), 1943– . II. Title. III. Series. [DNLM: 1. Photoreceptors – Physiology. 2. Vision – Physiology. WL 102.9 F299p]

QP481.F35 599.01′823 81-24209
ISBN 0 521 24433 1 hard covers AACR2
ISBN 0 521 28684 0 paperback

CONTENTS

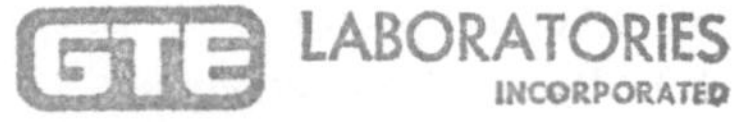

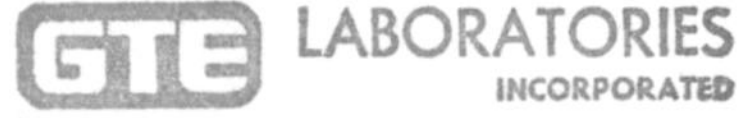
LABORATORIES
INCORPORATED

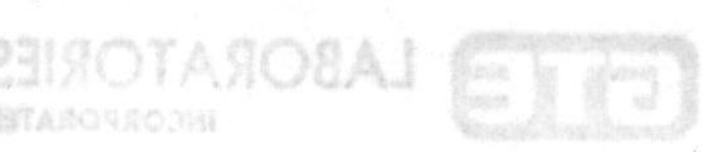

FOREWORD

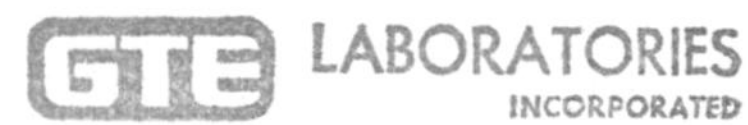

The origins of this series were a number of discussions in the Education Committee and in the Council of the International Union of Pure and Applied Biophysics (IUPAB). The subject of the discussions was the writing of a textbook in biophysics; the driving force behind the talks was Professor Aharon Katchalsky, first while he was president of the Union, and later as the honorary vice-president.

As discussions progressed, the concept of a unified text was gradually replaced by that of a series of short inexpensive volumes, each devoted to a single topic. It was felt that this format would be more flexible and more suitable in light of the rapid advances in many areas of biophysics at present. Instructors can use the volumes in various combinations according to the needs of their courses; new volumes can be issued as new fields become important and as current texts become obsolete.

The International Union of Pure and Applied Biophysics was motivated to participate in the publication of such a series for two reasons. First, the Union is in a position to give advice on the need for texts in various areas. Second, and even more important, it can help in the search for authors who have both the specific scientific background and the breadth of vision needed to organize the knowledge in their fields in a useful and lasting way.

The texts are designed for students in the last years of the standard university curriculum and for Ph.D. and M.D. candidates taking advanced courses. They should also provide a suitable introduction for someone about to begin research in a particular field of biophysics. The Union is pleased to collaborate with the Cambridge University Press in making these texts available to students and scientists throughout the world.

Franklin Hutchinson, Yale University
Watson Fuller, University of Keele
Lorin J. Mullins, University of Maryland
Raimundo Villegas, IVIC, Caracas
Editors

PREFACE

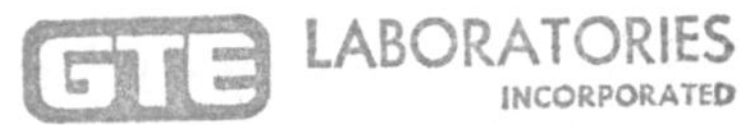

Research on photoreceptors has progressed at an ever-increasing pace making it very difficult for the nonexpert to keep abreast of new discoveries. The problem is compounded because interrelated advances are being made in the areas of morphology, biochemistry, and physiology. There is no paucity of excellent reviews addressed to experts within the field. Surprisingly, no analogous book or summaries yet exist for students or investigators who are new to this field. Our book is intended to fill this void. Specifically, its aim is to provide the novice with an integrated and up-to-date introduction to the role of photoreceptors in vision.

This book was written for an audience with at least a college-level knowledge of cell biology, biochemistry, physical chemistry, neurobiology, and physics. For anyone with this background, the book is self-contained. Others may need to consult a first-level text in their particular area of deficiency. Among the many excellent texts currently available, the following may serve as useful references: *Biochemistry,* A. L. Lehninger; *Biochemistry,* L. Stryer; *The Physiology of Excitable Cells,* D. J. Aidley; *From Neuron to Brain,* S. W. Kuffler and J. G. Nicholls; *Physical Biochemistry,* K. E. van Holde; *Optical Methods in Biology,* E. M. Slayter.

The material in this book is organized along two topical lines. First, having described the physical parameters of light in Chapter 1, we proceed in subsequent chapters to describe the mechanisms by which photoreceptors extract information about each parameter. The mechanisms exhibit varying complexity, and the length of their treatment varies accordingly. Whereas one chapter is sufficient for the discussion of one mechanism, several chapters are required for another. Second, the text is mainly organized by discipline, following the general sequence of cellular morphology (Chapters 2 and 3), visual pigment chemistry (Chapters 4–6), and receptor physiology (Chapters 7–12). This sequence of presentation naturally complements the description of the mechanisms for the detection of the physical parameters of light.

We regard our book as a "stepping stone" into the vast and exciting (perhaps sometimes baffling) scientific literature of the field, and as such we liberally used references. With the material in this book as background, the reader should be able to handle most, if not all, of the original articles. Because comparative physiology is an instructive way to study basic biological problems, we tried to give equal emphasis to both vertebrate and invertebrate receptors. However, a completely balanced presentation was not attempted, nor could it have been achieved, because vertebrates and invertebrates are not equally favored preparations for all studies. For example, the small number of photoreceptors in many invertebrate eyes precludes their use for most biochemical analyses. In order to make the book tractable, it was important to limit its length. Unfortunately, this required the omission of many interesting topics (experimental techniques, photoreceptor optics other than absorption, physiology of synaptic transmission) and limited the discussion of other issues (membrane biochemistry, color vision, psychophysics of threshold phenomenon, extracellularly recorded potentials such as the electroretinogram). We hope that through this book our readers will achieve sufficient expertise and enthusiasm to research the omitted topics on their own. Our ultimate aim in writing this text will then have been attained.

In a search for more complete understanding of basic cellular processes, modern research increasingly investigates cell function on the molecular level. In an active research area, such as the molecular basis of photoreceptor function, progress is often rapid and ideas are in a constant state of flux. The reader should be aware that the interpretation of the molecular models of visual excitation and adaptation in Chapters 11 and 12 may change drastically with new findings. Such revisions of interpretation are unlikely to occur for any of the earlier chapters.

Our way of looking at the biological universe was inevitably shaped by our teachers and colleagues. We can see their influences throughout the pages of this book. We thank them for their patience and counsel over the years. Our thanks also to E. F. MacNichol, Jr., F. I. Harosi, A. Kropf, L. E. Lipetz, J. S. Levine, S. C. Chamberlain, D. W. Corson, and S. Levy, who made many thoughtful suggestions throughout the gestation of this book. Alan Fein thanks the Neurobiology Unit of the Hebrew University of Jerusalem for their hospitality while this book was in preparation.

A. F.
E. Z. S.

Woods Hole
October, 1981

1 Vision and light

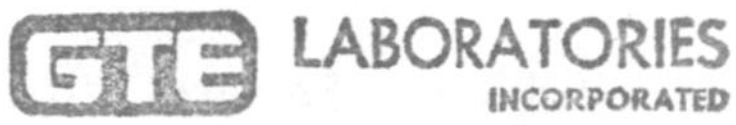

1.1 Vision as information processing

Vision is one of the major senses, sometimes the primary one, with which organisms perceive and interpret their surroundings. The visual process extracts "information" from the light that objects reflect to the eye, thereby supplying vital data for an organism's survival. Viewing the world comes so naturally to most of us that we do not consciously think about the kinds of visual information our brain processes. Suppose the reader were on a bird-watching expedition and someone nearby were to observe an unidentified warbler. The reader might ask: Where is it located? How fast is it moving? What color is it? How large is it? The answers to these kinds of questions are the types of information vision provides us continuously throughout our daily life. The type of information extracted from the environment depends on the specific needs of each organism. For example, some do not need to detect color and are therefore color blind, but others sense features that we humans cannot see. The initial steps of vision are accomplished by specialized neurons, called *photoreceptors*, which absorb light and generate neural signals. These signals pass along and through several levels of higher-order neurons where they undergo extensive processing before eventually transmitting their encoded information to the brain of the organism. It is this pathway of information processing that constitutes vision and differentiates it from photosynthesis and related processes that are similarly initiated by light absorption.

Before a serious discussion of the role of photoreceptors in vision can begin, the nature of the stimulus, which triggers the entire visual process, must be considered. Therefore, this chapter will focus on the physical parameters that characterize light.

1.2 Physical characteristics of light

Our earth is continuously bathed in a sea of electromagnetic radiation, which is almost exclusively generated by the sun. The spec-

Table 1.1. *Spectral distribution of sunlight incident on earth's atmosphere*

Spectral Region	Wavelength (nm)	Incident energy flux density ($\mu W\ cm^{-2}$)	Incident energy (%)
γ-Rays, X-rays, vacuum ultraviolet	<200	0.136	0.1
Far and near ultraviolet	200–400	16.2	11.9
Visible light	400–700	49.0	36.0
Near infrared	700–1000	32.6	24.0
Far infrared, radar, radio waves	>1000	38.1	28.0

Source: Seliger and McElroy, 1965.

trum of this radiation has no definite beginning or end and encompasses rays with greatly varying wavelengths. Only a relatively very narrow region of the wide continuum is detectable by the eyes of living organisms. We call the electromagnetic waves within that region "light." The visible spectrum's limits are defined in terms of human sensitivity. If the limits are arbitrarily taken to be the wavelengths at which human sensitivity drops to 1% of its maximum value, then the lower and upper bounds correspond to about 430 and 690 nm, respectively. In most of us, the lower limit is set by the lens of the eye, which strongly absorbs the near ultraviolet. If the lens is removed, as in corrective surgery for cataracts, the lower limit of the visible spectrum shifts below 350 nm (Wald, 1945). A less anthropocentric lower limit would be about 300 nm if insect vision were considered, and if fish were also included, the upper limit would extend to about 725 nm.

The visible spectrum corresponds to the most intense region of the solar spectrum (see Table 1.1). Light comprises 36% of the total solar energy incident on our planet. No other comparably wide spectral region, measured in wavelengths, contains as much energy.

Light, just as all other electromagnetic radiation, consists of oscillating electric and magnetic fields that are mutually perpendicular to each other. The properties of these fields can be described by five parameters, which completely characterize light and which are illustrated in Figure 1.1 for monochromatic plane waves. The five parameters are: wavelength, amplitude of the electric field, direction of travel, electric field orientation, and relative phase. Note that the magnetic field is not

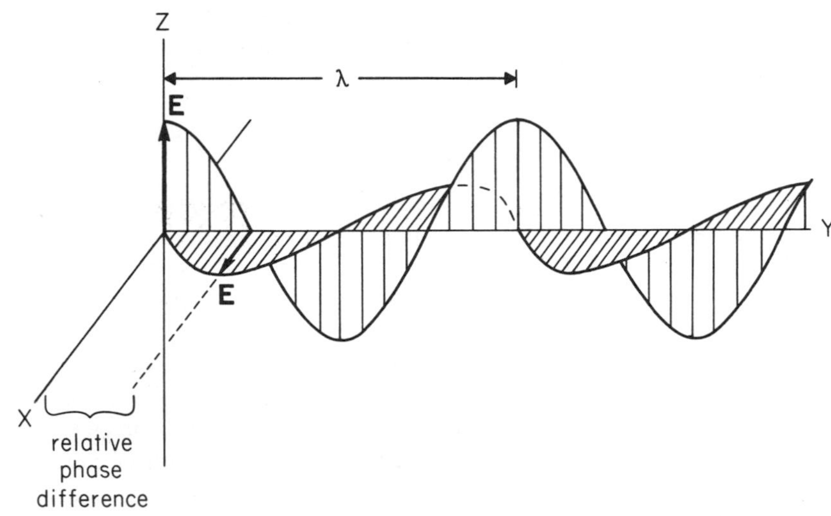

Figure 1.1. Two plane waves, illustrating the five parameters commonly employed for characterizing light waves. Both waves propagate in the same direction along the *y*-axis and both are of the same wavelength λ. Note that the electric field vectors **E**, whose magnitudes represent the waves' amplitudes at any given instant, are always perpendicular to the direction of propagation. The waves do not oscillate in unison but are out of phase by a quarter of a wavelength. Both waves are linearly polarized, so that their electric field vectors lie either within the *xy*- or the *yz*-plane.

illustrated in Figure 1.1. Its presence is ignored, because knowing the electric field's parameters completely specifies the magnetic field and because light's interaction with matter primarily involves the electric field.

The first parameter, wavelength, is the distance a wave front travels in the time its electric field oscillates through one cycle. For any medium, the product between wavelength and frequency is a constant and is equal to the speed of light.

Though it is a fundamental parameter, the amplitude of the electric field of a light beam is not a directly measurable quantity. However, the energy content of the light beam, to which it is related, can be directly measured; the relationship is such that the square of the maximal amplitude of the electric field is directly proportional to the beam's energy flux density (energy per unit time per unit area). Because the internationally accepted unit of energy is the joule, energy flux densities are expressed in units of joule second^{-1}-centimeter^{-2}, or more commonly in units of watt centimeter^{-2} (1 W = 1 J sec^{-1}). As is well known, light's energy is quantized into photons, that is into packets, whose energy is given by

$$\text{Energy} = hf = hc/\lambda, \tag{1.1}$$

where f is the frequency, λ the wavelength, c the velocity of light, and h Planck's constant. The energy and photon content of a light beam can be readily interconverted using Equation (1.1). The use of the term *intensity* to denote the energy content of a stimulus, whether it be delivered per unit time, per unit area, or per unit solid angle, is so embedded in the vision literature that it will be used throughout this book when referring to the amplitude or strength of the stimulus. The reader should note, however, that the most recent Système International d'Unités defines intensity as the energy emitted by a source per unit time per unit solid angle.

The electric field vector is constrained to lie within a plane, which is perpendicular to the direction of propagation and which is the xz-plane in Figure 1.1. Within that plane, the electric field vector can assume any orientation. Figure 1.1 illustrates two of the infinitely many possible orientations within the xz-plane. The electric field **E** of one of the waves is parallel to the z-axis and that of the other is parallel to the x-axis. Each of these waves is said to be *linearly polarized*, because the orientation of its **E**-vector is invariant with time.

The last of the aforementioned parameters, relative phase, relates a wave's oscillations to a spatial or temporal reference point. With respect to each other, the two waves of Figure 1.1 are out of phase by a quarter of a wavelength. When plane waves are superimposed, their relative phases can produce destructive or constructive interference, meaning that the amplitude of the final wave varies anywhere between zero and the linear sum of the individual amplitudes.

It is important to realize that monochromatic plane waves are idealized representations, approximated only within the laboratory through the use of lasers. Natural light is equivalent to a superposition of many plane waves, each with its own wavelength, intensity, electric field orientation, relative phase, and direction of propagation. The heterogenous nature of light makes its representation by a single wavelength, with a given electric field orientation or a specific relative phase, impossible. As a result, these parameters are replaced by the related terms of spectral composition, degree of polarization, and degree of coherence.

All the physical parameters of light are potentially capable of providing information to an organism about its surroundings. Visually sensitive organisms may detect some of these parameters, with sensitivity to any one of them being highly variable among species. As will be discussed in the next section, humans are one of the many organisms that make only partial use of all the available visual information.

1.3 Human visual system and natural illumination

The human visual system can be used to illustrate how one type of visual system has adapted to and been able to extract visual information from its environment. In this context, it is appropriate to consider the range of values for each of light's parameters in the natural environment and the corresponding range for human perception.

An important point, which will remain relevant for the remainder of this book, needs to be stressed here. The attributes of an entire visual system do not necessarily reflect the properties of its photoreceptors. Though the latter certainly play a dominant role, what we and other organisms "see" also depends on signal processing by higher-order neurons. For humans, the actual sensation of seeing ultimately involves cells in the visual cortex, far removed from the receptors. Blind people, for example, "see" if their cortical cells are artificially stimulated with electrodes. The popular adage of "seeing with one's eyes" is a poetic simplification.

1.3.1 Direction of propagation

Whether it is scattered, reflected, or refracted, light reaches an organism from all directions. It is desirable, therefore, to be able to monitor one's environment over as large a solid angle as possible. Ideally, the visual field should be the maximum 360°. Except for some unicellular organisms this optimal visual field is rarely realized. For most organisms, a large visual field is useless if shapes within it cannot be discerned; if, say, a potential predator cannot be discriminated from a harmless plant. Partly for this reason, arrays of photoreceptors are found in *image-forming structures* called *eyes*. By processing the signals emanating from the receptor array, organisms are able to discriminate among objects within their visual field. Such processing allows humans to perform a variety of visual tasks, such as reading the words of this sentence. The performance of any optical instrument, such as an eye, can be measured by its ability to resolve spatial detail. This ability is commonly called *spatial resolution* and will be discussed further in Section 2.4.

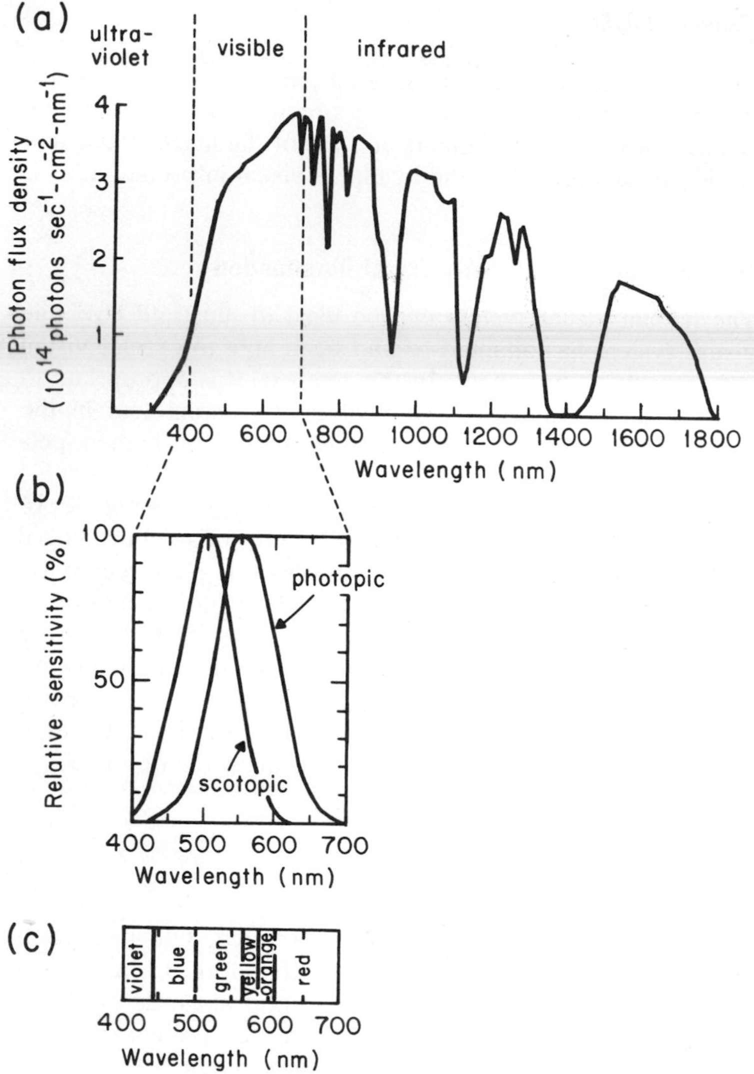

Figure 1.2. (*a*) Spectral distribution of sunlight, as measured at the surface of the earth on a cloudless day, with the sun's elevation 30° above the horizon. On integrating the area beneath the curve, the flux density of all the incident photons is about 10^{17} photons cm^{-2}-sec^{-1} within the visible range (400–700 nm). (After Seliger, 1977.) (*b*) Spectral sensitivity of the normal human eye when ambient light intensities are dim (dark-adapted eye or scotopic vision) or bright (light-adapted eye or photopic vision). The curves are the internationally recognized standards of the Commission Internationale de l'Eclairage (CIE). (After LeGrand, 1957.) (*c*) Distribution of colors within the visible spectrum as seen by humans. For individuals with normal color vision, variability in the location of the transition zones between adjacent colors is less than 10 nm. (After LeGrand, 1957.)

1.3.2 Spectral composition

Figure 1.2*a* illustrates the spectral distribution of sunlight throughout the visible and infrared spectrum. Note that the spectrum is plotted in terms of photons and could be easily converted to an energy spectrum by the use of Equation (1.1). The relative contribution of specific spectral regions to the overall spectrum varies with the two different plots. For example, the relative contribution of short wavelengths is greater with an energy plot because the energy of a photon is inversely proportional to its wavelength.

To humans, sunlight's spectral composition appears white. The wide variety of colors we encounter in nature is due to the modification of this spectral composition by molecules that either scatter or absorb light. The perceived hue generally depends on the wavelength(s) at which photon flux density is the largest. For example, the sky away from the sun appears blue because atmospheric molecules preferentially scatter shorter wavelengths, causing the photon flux density of skylight to peak at about 450 nm (McFarland and Munz, 1975). Correspondingly, tree leaves are green because their chlorophylls preferentially absorb photons in the red and blue end of the spectrum and reflect or transmit the unabsorbed green light. Similar effects are produced when light is transmitted through pigmented media, such as oceans, lakes, and colored filters, each containing its unique blend of light-absorbing pigments. It is likely that natural selection has favored organisms whose spectral sensitivities match the spectral distribution of their habitat. In humans, spectral sensitivity peaks at 550 nm (green region) under bright light conditions and at 500 nm (blue-green region) with very dim light (Figures 1.2*b* and *c*). As will be discussed later, we perceive colors only if the light intensities are sufficiently bright to stimulate our cones.

1.3.3 Intensity

Intensities normally encountered in nature can vary by a factor of 10^{15} (Table 1.2). Remarkably, the human visual system functions over most of this range; that is, it responds to light over a range of 10^{12}, but the response is not always instantaneous. For any ambient background intensity, the range over which humans can instantaneously respond is only about 10^{3}. As background intensities increase or decrease, visual sensitivity is commensurately altered, shifting the instantaneously available range up or down the intensity scale. This shift takes minutes or tens of minutes and is mediated primarily by biochemical reactions within the receptors. Variation of visual sensi-

Table 1.2. *Range of light intensities naturally encountered and the range of human vision*

Photic conditions	Energy flux density at the earth's surface (log μW cm^{-2})[a]	Range of human vision for stated energy flux density at retina	
		} solar burn of the retina[d]	
	7		
	6		
Bright June day[b]	5		
	4		photopic
	3		
	2	cone range[d]	
End of twilight[b]	1		
Full moon[b]	0		
	−1		
	−2		
	−3		mesopic
	−4	rod range[d]	
	−5		
	−6		
	−7		scotopic
Darkest night sky[c]	−8		
	−9		

[a] On this logarithmic scale, 10^6 μW cm^{-2} corresponds to 6, 1 μW cm^{-2} corresponds to 0, and so forth.
[b] From Seliger and McElroy, 1965.
[c] From Pirenne, 1962.
[d] From Weale, 1961; stimulus a short flash of white light.

tivity with light intensity is called *adaptation* and is the process responsible for the large visual ranges of humans and of other organisms.

In a discussion of visual range, the use of scientific notation for specifying intensities becomes bulky. Therefore, visual physiologists express relative intensity values on a logarithmic scale, where each log unit refers to a tenfold increase in intensity. Such a scale is used in Table 1.2. To appreciate the range of human vision, one should remember that photographic emulsions used in camera films function over a maximum range of only 10^3, or 3 log units. They cannot adapt.

Another remarkable fact about the human visual system is that with its system of rod photoreceptors it is one of the most sensitive photon detectors. The absorption of a single photon is sufficient to excite a rod (Chapter 9). As Table 1.2 illustrates, we refer to *scotopic, photopic,* and *mesopic* vision whenever we use our rods, cones, or a combination of the two sets of receptors, respectively.

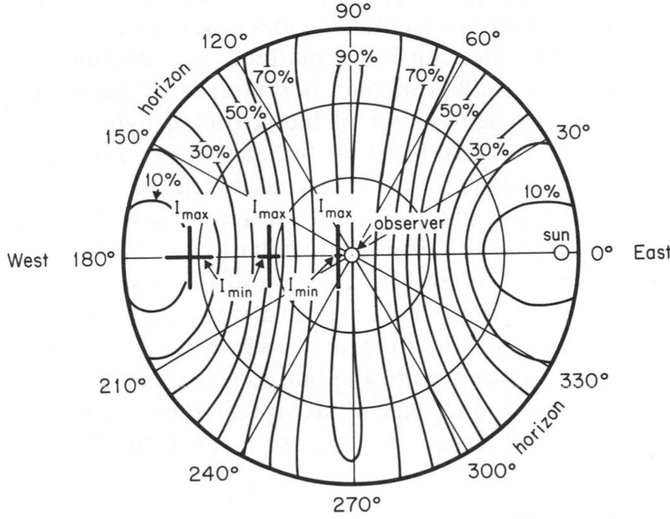

Figure 1.3. Polarization of the sky at dawn. The polar graph is a two-dimensional representation of the celestial hemisphere, with the sun near the horizon and the observer at the center of the graph, directly below the zenith. Contours connect points with an equal degree of polarization, where degree of polarization is given in percents and is defined as $[(I_{max} - I_{min})/(I_{max} + I_{min})]100$. Maximum intensity I_{max}, refers to the light intensity along the axis of polarization. Perpendicular to this axis is the direction of the minimum intensity I_{min}. The orientation and relative intensities of I_{max} and I_{min} are shown for selected points on the east–west meridian. Polarization is always maximum along an arc that is traced out by the plane, which includes the observer and is perpendicular to the sun's direction. The degree of polarization gradually decreases as the point being observed moves toward or away from the sun. The polarization axis is easily determined for any point in the sky because it is always perpendicular to the plane of the triangle formed by the observer, the sun, and the observed point in the sky. (After Wehner, 1976.)

1.3.4 Degree of polarization

The notion that polarized light is a common natural phenomenon comes as a surprise to most of us. Our surprise, of course, is a reflection of our inability to detect polarized light. Under ideal conditions, some humans can observe a polarization-induced visual phenomenon, the so-called Haidinger's brush effect (Brindley, 1970), but its detection is so rare that our generalization about human blindness to polarization is valid. Although our insensitivity is shared by all vertebrates, many invertebrates (cephalopods and insects being the best-known examples) possess highly developed polarization sensitivity.

Light radiated by the sun is unpolarized. In traveling through the earth's atmosphere, however, light is scattered by the air molecules, causing the electric field vector of the scattered light to vibrate in a certain direction at each point in the sky. Only *scattered* light is polarized, *direct* sunlight is not. When looking at the sky, the degree of polarization is always greatest along an arc, which, forming a plane with the observer on earth, is perpendicular to the sun's direction. This arc also corresponds to the bluest region of the sky. When the sun is near the horizon, the arc of maximal polarization passes directly overhead (Figure 1.3). When the sun reaches a position overhead, the arc of maximal polarization moves to the horizon. Skylight polarization can be a useful visual cue and, indeed, as von Frisch (1967) demonstrated in his now classic experiments, bees use it for navigational purposes.

1.3.5 Degree of coherence

Visual systems, in general, are incapable of detecting incident light's relative phase for the purpose of extracting information about the environment. For example, humans could not perceive the phase differences of the two monochromatic waves of Figure 1.1. Nevertheless, under certain conditions, relative phase becomes a major factor in vision because ocular structures can give rise to diffraction effects. For example, human visual acuity is almost limited by the diffraction effects of the pupil when it contracts to a minimal diameter of 2 mm with bright lights. Diffraction considerations are even more important in the compound eyes of insects because insect facets are much smaller than the human pupil.

1.4 Summary

Direction of propagation, spectral composition, intensity, degree of polarization, and degree of coherence are the characteristic parameters of light that, in principle, could be sensed by light detectors. Organisms use their sensory modalities to learn about their external world; hence it is not surprising that visual systems in general have developed the capacity to detect some of these parameters. Specifically, organisms can resolve objects in their visual field, and they are sensitive to the spectral composition, intensity, and degree of polarization of light.

2 Ocular organization

Photoreceptors are often found in image-forming structures called *eyes*. Ocular organization is such that photoreceptors are rarely the first cells to be encountered by incident light. Rather, light must pass through several cell layers and perhaps over centimeter-long distances before it finally reaches the receptors. Transmission through these accessory cells and structures can substantially modify the spectral composition, degree of polarization, and intensity of the incident light. As already mentioned in Chapter 1, the lens is the limiting factor in the detection of short-wavelength light in humans. To appreciate fully the constraints that ocular structures place on image formation, the salient features of some common eyes will be considered in this chapter. The major emphasis will be on a consideration of how ocular organization constrains the spatial resolution of visual systems.

2.1 Simple eyes

The tendency among physiologists is to call eyes either *simple* or *complex* on the basis of their capability to form an image. The dividing line is rather hazy because the quality of image formation varies greatly. As a result, simple eyes can display a wide range of functional and anatomical complexity: from an unorganized group of receptors (such as the ventral photoreceptors of *Limulus polyphemus*), to a cup-shaped organ where receptors line the inner surface (as in some snails), and, finally, to a well-developed ocellus that contains a lens capable of some crude image formation (as in some spiders and insects). The most rudimentary eyes completely lack image formation. Nevertheless, their receptors may resemble the receptors of more complex eyes on the physiological and biochemical level. As a result, such photoreceptors can be extremely useful preparations for visual studies, especially if their cell bodies are exceptionally large, which facilitates intracellular electrophysiological recording.

2.2 Complex eyes

Image formation attained its highest level among vertebrates (all classes), arthropods (most classes), mollusks (mainly the class of cephalopods), and annelid worms (solely confined to a single family, the alciopids; see Wald and Rayport, 1977). Their complex eyes can be conveniently sorted into three groups: vertebrate, compound, and cephalopod eyes.

2.2.1 Vertebrate eye

Basic anatomy. All vertebrates possess the same basic eye structure, illustrated in Figure 2.1*a*. The vertebrate eye is essentially a fluid-filled sac bounded by three concentric layers of tissue. The outermost layer is composed of a tough, collagenous material, which, in conjunction with the pressure of the intraocular fluid, gives the eye its overall shape. Except for its most anterior region, the outer layer is opaque and is known as the *sclera,* the "white of the eye." At the globe's anterior, the outer layer is transparent and is called the *cornea*. Adjacent and interior to the sclera is a second tissue layer, the *uvea,* whose three regional differentiations are called the *choroid,* the *ciliary body,* and the *iris*. The third and innermost layer is the *retina* (Figure 2.1*b*), composed of the *pigment epithelium* and the *neural retina*. A light-transparent fluid occupies the bulk of the eye's volume.

Image formation. The cornea and lens are the structures that form the optical images on the back of the retina. For terrestrial animals, most of the refraction occurs at the cornea, or, more precisely, at the air–corneal interface, where the refractive index differential, the actual source of ray "bending," is greater than at the aqueous-humor–lens interface. Reducing the eye's focal length so that an image remains in focus at the retinal plane is called *accommodation* and, in terrestrial animals, is mainly accomplished by an increase in the lens's curvature. The focal length of the cornea–lens combination is 17 mm when an adult with normal vision views objects more than 3 m away. For near vision, the focal length decreases to 14 mm. By varying the pupillary area, the iris regulates the amount of light reaching the retina and hence controls image brightness.

Retina. The neural retina consists of several types of glial cells and of six types of neurons, which include the photoreceptors. It is several hundred microns thick, equivalent to the thickness of a sheet of paper, and is essentially avascular. Retinal cells receive nourishment partly

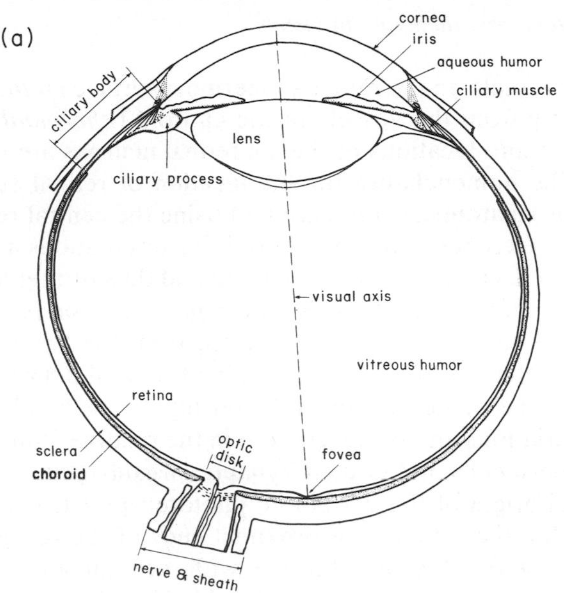

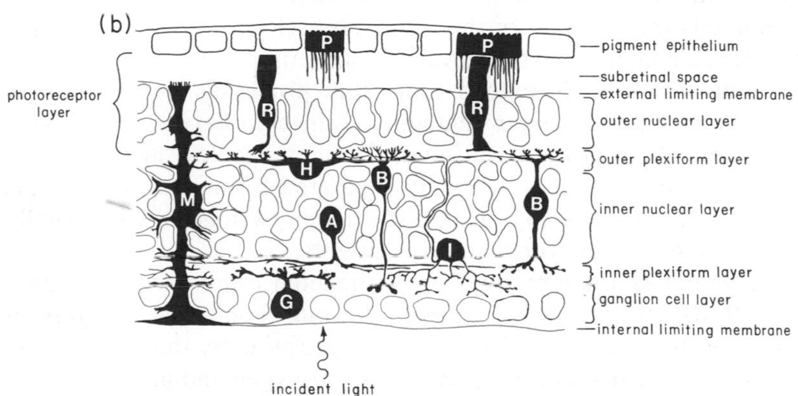

Figure 2.1. The vertebrate eye. (*a*) Horizontal cross section of a human right eye, showing major structures. Note that the optic disk is located nasally to the fovea, so that its corresponding blindspot, after taking into account the inverting properties of the lens, falls to the right of the point of fixation. (After Walls, 1942.) (*b*) Schematic drawing of a generalized vertebrate retina. The six types of retinal neurons are: receptors (R), horizontal cells (H), bipolar cells (B), amacrine cells (A), interplexiform cells (I), and ganglion cells (G). The cell bodies of these neurons form distinct layers: the outer nuclear layer, the inner nuclear layer, and the ganglion cell layer. Their synaptic processes are nearly exclusively found within the outer and inner plexiform layers. Only the predominant glial cell, the "Müller fiber" (M), is shown. Opposing the distal tips of the receptors are the cells of the pigment epithelium (P). (After Dowling, 1970.)

from the blood vessels on the retina's innermost surface (*retinal circulation*) and partly from the vessels of the choroid (*choroidal circulation*). The names and locations of the six retinal neurons are shown in Figure 2.1*b*. The nomenclature for the location of retinal structures follows the neuroanatomical convention of using the central regions of the brain as the reference point for determining orientations and directions. A structure located nearer to the brain and thus further along the path of sensory information flow is called *proximal,* or *inner.* Conversely, a retinal structure furthest removed from the brain is called *distal,* or *outer.* Retinal neurons are confined to well-defined layers, which maintain the same relative relationship to each other in all vertebrates. Variations among species are in the relative number, size, and shape of these cells and in their synaptic organization.

The epithelial origin of the vertebrate photoreceptor is revealed by its location within the retina. The proximal ends of the receptors are firmly embedded within the neural tissue, with receptor somas forming the outer nuclear layer. The receptors' distal half, including the visual-pigment-containing *outer segment,* are essentially unsupported as they protrude into the extracellular fluid of the subretinal space. The *subretinal space* is the remnant of the brain ventricle that collapsed during neural development. Also bordering the subretinal space is the pigment epithelium, whose cells extend long, thin processes that intimately ensheath the opposing outer segments. Adhesion between the retina and the epithelium is quite variable. In many species, including primates, the two layers can be easily separated from each other. This property is of relevance to biochemists and physiologists, who usually require isolated retinas for their experiments.

The pigment epithelium plays a multifaceted role in receptor function. With its light-absorbing *pigment granules* containing *melanin,* it absorbs nearly all the light that escapes absorption by the photoreceptors. It is an intermediary in the delivery of oxygen and nutrients from the choroidal circulation. Furthermore, it plays an active role in the continuous turnover of the outer segments, and in those amphibians capable of tissue regeneration, its cells can differentiate to replace lost retinal neurons (Reyer, 1977). So essential is the epithelium to the receptors that should their normal interaction be terminated either by physical separation (as in detached retinas) or by specific genetic defects (as in some forms of retinitis pigmentosa), receptor function can be seriously damaged, leading to receptor atrophy and, eventually, blindness.

Consequence of receptor location. The distal location of vertebrate photoreceptors has two characteristic consequences: degraded image formation and blindness at a specific region of the visual field. Image formation is degraded because light rays have to traverse the blood vessels and the neural layers before they can be detected by the receptors. Though retinal neurons, with the exception of receptors, do not absorb light, they scatter it because they, as most cells, are optically inhomogeneous. For example, in the 200-μm-thick turtle retina, scatter increases the initial diameter of a parallel beam from 8 to 50 μm at the outer segment level (or from 1 to 5 receptor diameters), thereby attenuating the light intensity in the center by more than tenfold (Baylor et al., 1971). Such scatter seriously impedes spatial resolution. An obvious way to overcome the problem would be to remove the intervening blood vessels and cells. This is indeed what happens in the vertebrate *fovea* (Figure 2.1*a*), found in primates and in some species of birds, but not in most vertebrates. Retinal thickness is drastically reduced as blood vessels and all the higher-order neurons are laterally displaced. Such a solution is so effective in reducing scatter that foveal acuity is even further increased by a tight packing of thin receptors, which, in humans, are exclusively cones. The human fovea is round, and with a diameter of 1.5 mm or 5° of visual angle, it occupies less than 0.1% of the entire retinal surface. As shown in Figure 2.1*a*, it is located on the very center of the visual axis so that whenever we fixate on an object, the object's image directly falls on the fovea.

Localized blindness is a consequence of the fact that the nerve fibers of the ganglion cells must pass out of the eye to reach other parts of the brain and so must displace receptors in the process. Their point of exit, which is also the passageway for blood vessels and for efferent fibers from the brain, is called the *optic disk* (Figure 2.1*a*). The field the optic disk subtends in visual space is called the *blindspot* and its size is about 7° in humans. The visual impediment caused by the blindspot is minimized in all animals by its shape and location (for comparative anatomy, see Walls, 1942). In animals such as primates, with frontal eyes and hence with large fields of binocular vision, the fields circumscribed by each spot fall within the binocular field so that part of the visual field of one eye overlaps the blindspot of the other. Although the blindspot could become a serious impediment in monocular individuals, its inconvenience is remarkably minimized: (1) by its location in a region of relatively low visual acuity and (2) by the unconscious rapid movements of the eye.

Photoreceptors. As will be discussed in Chapter 3, vertebrate photoreceptors can be classified as either rods or cones. The number of receptors per retina can be enormous; in humans, there are about 1.2×10^8 rods and 6×10^6 cones (Østerberg, 1935).

Receptor distribution varies across the hemispheric retinal surface of all animals, including humans (Østerberg, 1935). For example, rods are completely absent in the very center of the human fovea, within half a degree of the visual axis. In this region, the long, slender cones are packed into a density of about 1.5×10^5 mm^{-2}, with an interreceptor distance of 2.8 μm. Toward the periphery, rod and cone densities rapidly rise and fall, respectively, so that at angles greater than about 1° from the visual axis, rods outnumber cones at each retinal region, sometimes by as much as a factor of 30.

Retinal organization also varies in a characteristic manner for animals that have adapted to different photic environments. Specifically, the rod-to-cone ratio is much greater in nocturnal retinas than in diurnal or crepuscular ones. For example, the ratio is about 4000 for the nocturnal rat (LaVail, 1976*b*) but is 1 for frogs (Liebman and Entine, 1968), 15 for goldfish (Stell and Harosi, 1976), and 20 for humans (Østerberg, 1935). Retinas containing both rods and cones are said to be *duplex*. Though most animals possess duplex retinas, many fish, especially those living in deep waters, appear to lack cones (see compendium by Ali and Anctil, 1976). No organism with a pure cone retina is yet known, though the retinas of lizards and birds of prey come the closest. The correspondence between anatomical variation and photic preference was an early clue, recognized by the eminent nineteenth-century physiologist M. Schultze (1866), that rods are the primary receptors of dim-light vision and cones of bright-light vision.

2.2.2 Compound eye

Basic anatomy. Compound eyes consist of hundreds or thousands of nearly identical units called *ommatidia*. Each ommatidium is analogous to a vertebrate eye with its own refractile apparatus and its own "little retina" or *retinula* (see Figure 2.2). The refractile apparatus with its cornea and a "crystalline cone" is functionally analogous to the vertebrate cornea and lens. In insects, however, the structures do not absorb the near ultraviolet. (The crystalline cones are not and should not be confused with photoreceptors.) The repeat pattern of the ommatidial corneas gives rise to the faceted appearance of compound eyes. The facets are arranged in rows, and in cross section, they resemble polygons with from four to six sides. Beneath the crystalline cones, the ommatidia are cylindrical (about 50 μm wide and 500 μm long; these dimensions are variable among species), and their sides are lined with accessory cells, which are pigmented and which can potentially shield against light leakage between adjacent ommatidia. The degree of shielding is species-dependent and varies with the state of adaptation. The retinula consists of only a few photoreceptors (eight or more), called *retinular cells,* and only in a few genera (such as *Limulus*)

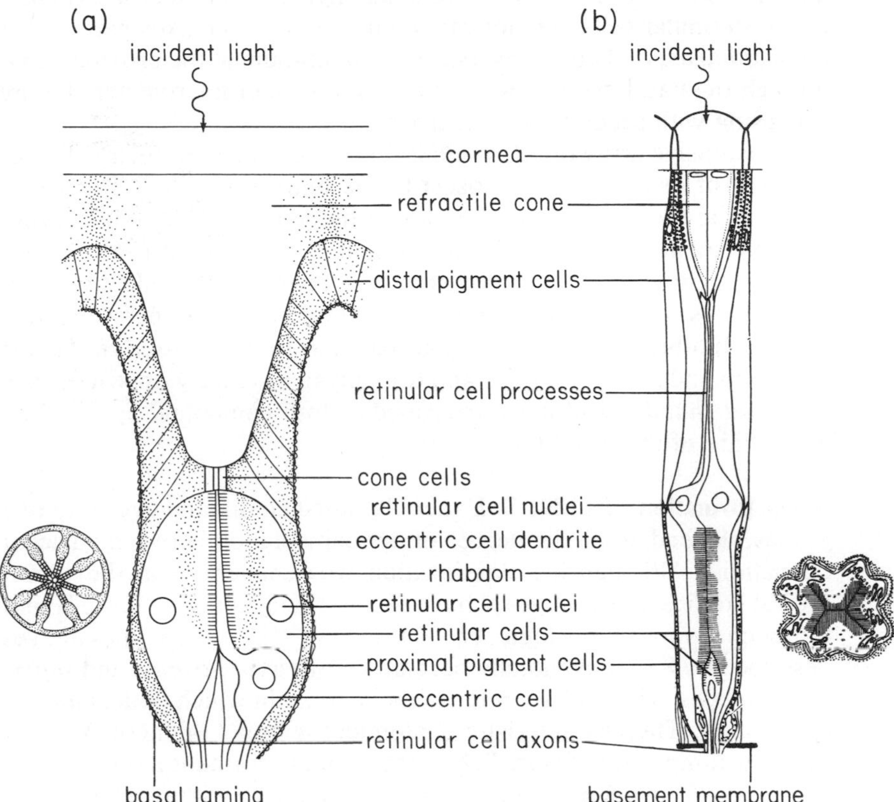

Figure 2.2. Anatomy of the ommatidia of superposition and apposition type compound eyes. Cross-sectional views are parallel to the ommatidial axis and for the inserts perpendicular to the ommatidial axis at the rhabdom regions. (*a*) The apposition-type lateral eye of *Limulus*. The entire ommatidium with its fused rhabdom is about 1 mm long, with the axial length of the cornea and crystalline cone together being about 650 μm. The rhabdom region spans about 180 μm. The ommatidial facets, which are flat and featureless, are about 200 μm in diameter. (After Fahrenbach, 1975.) (*b*) The superposition eye of skipper butterflies. The entire ommatidium with its fused rhabdom is 0.4–1.0 mm long, with the cornea and cone together being about 100 μm. The rhabdom region spans several hundred micrometers and is separated from the refractile cone by a nearly equally wide optically clear zone. Facet diameters are about 30 μm. (After Horridge et al., 1972.)

does it contain one or two additional higher-order neurons (Figure 2.2*a*). Retinular cells are elongated units whose long axes parallel the ommatidial axis. Their axons exit the ommatidium at the proximal end, through the basal membrane, and traverse tens of micrometers before synapsing with second-order neurons.

An extensive array of *microvilli* is formed by each retinular cell over that part of its cell surface closest to the ommatidial axis. The visual pigments are located within the plasma membrane of these microvilli. The microvilli of a receptor cell are collectively called *rhabdomere*, and the eight or more rhabdomeres of a retinula are collectively referred to as a *rhabdom*. Adjacent rhabdomeres are either separated from each other by large interstitial space, as in the *unfused rhabdoms* of diptera and hemiptera (flies and true bugs), or closely opposed, as in the *fused rhabdoms* of most arthropods. Both compound eyes in Figure 2.2 are of the fused type.

Image formation In 1891 S. Exner classified compound eyes into two groups, depending on the degree of optical isolation between adjacent ommatidia. Although his classification was challenged in the 1950s, critical studies in recent years have reconfirmed Exner's views. [For a thorough review of this topic, see Kunze (1979).] The two types of eyes described by Exner eventually became known as *apposition* and *superposition* eyes. Their names refer to the manner in which optical images are formed. The characteristic anatomical features of these types of eyes are compared in Figure 2.2 and their image formation is compared in Figure 2.3. In apposition eyes, the optical image within any ommatidium is formed by rays that have traversed only its own facet. The state of light or dark adaptation does not greatly affect the degree of screening in the ommatidial walls and hence does not substantially alter this condition of image formation. By contrast, in superposition eyes, the optical image is formed by rays that have traversed the facets of many, even hundreds, of adjacent ommatidia. The amount of light that can pass through the ommatidial walls of these eyes is dependent on the light-induced pigment migration. In bright light, when screening is maximal, their image formation approximates that observed in apposition eyes. As Goldsmith (1973) has pointed out, apposition eyes are characteristic of diurnal animals, and superposition eyes are distinctive of nocturnal animals. Therefore, he refers to these types of eyes as *photopic* and *scotopic*, respectively. Aside from their manner of image formation, the location of their rhabdoms is also characteristic. In apposition eyes, the distal tips of rhabdomeres are located near the apical portion of the crystalline cones (see Figure 2.2*a*), whereas in superposition eyes, a wide optically clear zone is interposed between

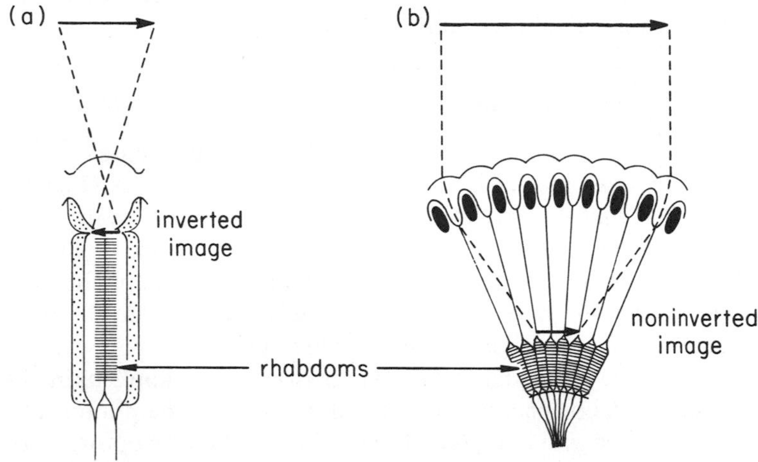

Figure 2.3. Optical image formation in compound eyes. (*a*) In apposition eyes such as *Limulus* (see Figure 2.2*a*), the inverted image is brought to a focus near the ends of the crystalline cones, at the distal tips of the retinular cells and rhabdoms. (*b*) In superposition eyes such as in skipper butterflies (see Figure 2.2*b*), the image is located far (100–200 μm) from the ends of the crystalline cones, although still at the distal tips of the rhabdoms. The real image is not inverted. Light adaptation displaces the screening pigments, so that light passage between adjacent ommatidia is reduced.

these structures (see Figure 2.2*b*). Only fused rhabdoms have been reported so far for superposition eyes.

Organisms with compound eyes are incapable of varying their focal length. However, accommodation by them is not as essential because their focal lengths are so short (e.g., focal length in the lateral eye of *Limulus* is 260 μm; Land, 1979) that objects a few centimeters away are effectively at infinity. It appears that, irrespective of the type of eye, optical images are in focus at or near the distal tips of the rhabdoms. In apposition eyes, the image is inverted, and in superposition ones, it is not (see Figure 2.3). Compound eyes use migrating screening pigments to regulate the amount of light reaching their receptors (see discussion in Chapter 8). In superposition eyes, these screening pigments are located between ommatidia and restrict light collection through adjacent facets. In apposition eyes, such as *Limulus*, light collection is primarily controlled by the constriction of pigmented cells that bridge the apical end of the crystalline cone with the distal tip of the rhabdom (Barlow et al., 1980). These cells are functional equivalents of the vertebrate pupil.

2.2.3 Cephalopod eye

The cephalopod eye appears to be a composite of the two complex eyes just discussed. Its refractile apparatus (Figure 2.4*a*) is similar to that of vertebrates, and its retina resembles the simplicity of insect retinulas. For the class of cephalopods, which include the nautiloids, octopuses, and squids, the squid eye is perhaps the best characterized. Squids may possess the largest eyes of any living creature. Deep-sea–dwelling giant squids, which are sometimes captured, have eyes that may be as large as 40 cm in diameter (Akimushkin, 1965). The squid retina consists of one type of neural cell, the photoreceptor, and two types of glial cells (see Figure 2.4*b*). Photoreceptors make up the bulk of the cellular volume and span the entire thickness of the retina (500 μm). They are bipolar neurons, whose long distal segments are directed toward the lens and account for more than half of the retinal thickness. Although all squid receptors are thought to be identical in function, there is a large variation in their cross section. It is not yet clear whether this variation is from the presence of several discrete types of cells (such as rods and cones in vertebrates) or from a continuous distribution in the size of one receptor type. Distal segments are richly covered with the microvilli that contain the visual pigments. Within any receptor, the microvilli are parallel to each other but are perpendicular to the microvilli of adjoining neighbors (Figure 2.4*c*).

Image formation in cephalopods is the same as in vertebrates. The only essential difference being that in cephalopods the visual pigment-containing distal segments are the first retinal structures to be encountered by the incident light (Figure 2.4*b*). The effect of this is that light scatter is greatly reduced and blindspots are absent.

2.3 Extraretinal photoreceptors

Photoreceptors need not exist exclusively within eyes or retinas; their occurrence in other locations is a common biological phenomenon. The best-known examples include: (1) discrete neurons of the abdominal ganglia in sea hare (*Aplysia californica*) and in crayfish (Arvanitaki and Chalazonitis, 1961; Larimer et al., 1966); (2) the isolated sphincter muscle of the iris in amphibians and some mammals (Barr and Alpern, 1963; Bito and Turansky, 1975); and (3) the discrete neurons of the pineal system found in most vertebrates (Hamasaki and Eder, 1977). These receptors may not completely resemble visual

(a)

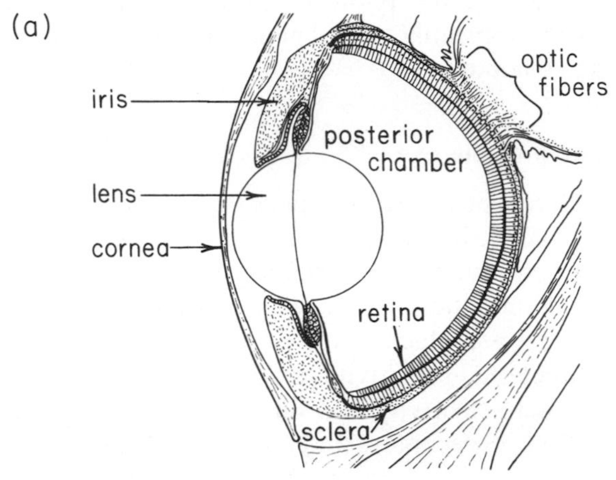

(b)

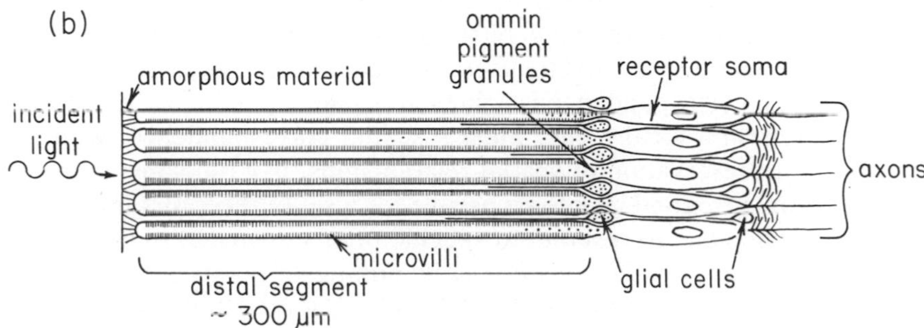

(c)

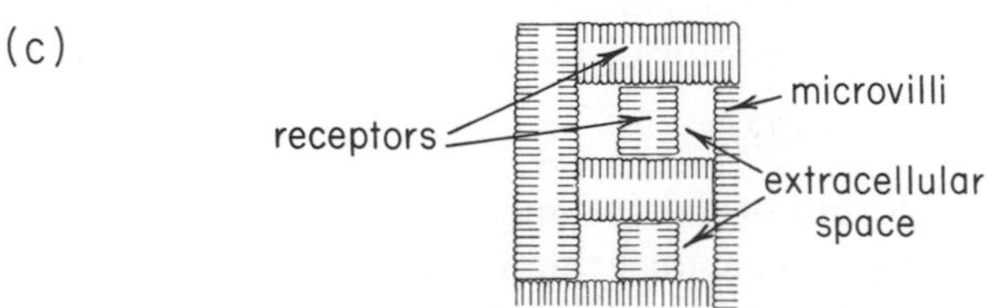

Figure 2.4. The cephalopod eye. (*a*) Cross section through the squid eye with identification of its major structures. (After Williams, 1909.) (*b*) A schematic drawing showing the three principal cells of the squid retina. Note that, in contrast to vertebrates, incident light in cephalopods encounters the photoreceptors before it traverses the retina. (After Zonana, 1961; Cohen, 1973.) (*c*) Receptors in cross section at the level of their distal segments. (After Zonana, 1961.)

photoreceptors. For example, the photoreceptors of the abdominal ganglia of *Aplysia* lack rhodopsinlike visual pigments and are relatively insensitive to light (see Chapter 11).

2.4 Spatial resolution of the eye

Individual photoreceptors are very poor detectors of the direction of incident light. That is, if a single photoreceptor were removed from an eye and placed on a surface, it would respond almost equally well to all directions of illumination. However, it could be made preferentially sensitive with proper placement of screening pigments. In essence, this is how directional sensitivity is achieved by simple eyes. To achieve the directional sensitivity and fine resolution of complex eyes, a large number of photoreceptors and an image-forming lens are necessary.

The lens, or its refractile equivalent, is essential because light rays from a point source ordinarily travel in all directions. Though they have the same origin in space, these rays strike a surface at various angles. A lens differentially refracts all the rays originating from a specific point in space and focuses them back into a single spot. Thus a one-to-one correspondence is achieved between points in a visual field and points in a focal plane. Such a spatial correspondence, with the attendant preservation of spatial relationships, is a fundamental property of all lenses and makes it possible for a set of receptors positioned in the focal plane to respond to specific points in space. In this sense, each photoreceptor is sensitive to its conjugate points in space. The angle by which the conjugate points of adjacent receptors are separated relates to spatial resolution, or acuity. The angle that each receptor subtends by itself (*acceptance angle*) depends on receptor size, and the angle that a visual system can potentially resolve (*inter-receptor angle*) depends on inter-receptor distance. Either angle is given by

$$\text{angle} = 2 \tan^{-1}(d/2f) \qquad (2.1)$$

where f is the focal length of the eye and d is either the inter-receptor distance (when the inter-receptor angle is calculated) or the effective diameter of the visual pigment-containing organelle (when the acceptance angle is being determined).

Excitation of an individual receptor is insufficient for resolving objects in visual space. An organism must also sense whether or not neighboring cells are excited. *Resolution requires the differential excitation of many neighboring receptors.*

To illustrate these simple concepts consider a 35-mm camera, whose focal length is 50 mm and which is loaded with a film containing 1-μm-sized silver halide crystals (a common size). Because the crystals are independent, light-absorbing units, they are analogous to receptor cells. Using Equation (2.1), the angle subtended by each halide crystal can be calculated to be about 0.0001°, or 3 sec of arc. This is also the camera's ultimate resolution because the center-to-center distance between closely packed crystals is comparable to crystal size. Visual systems rarely, if ever, achieve such a resolution.

Many factors besides the interreceptor angle contribute to the spatial resolution of visual systems. These additional factors are:

a. Optical limitations. Diffraction, scatter, and the host of imperfections that are inherent properties of lenses all degrade the one-to-one correspondence between image and object space.
b. Signal summation by the visual system. Receptor signals can be pooled by higher-order neurons so that the final resolving power of a visual system is worse than if it were solely determined by receptor density alone (see Section 2.4.1).
c. Light intensity. For optimum resolution, the illumination must be sufficiently intense to ensure that photons are absorbed by all the illuminated receptors. Of course, intensity can further alter resolution by its effect on signal summation (see b) and screening-pigment migration (Chapter 8).

The previous discussion presented the most important factors and principles of spatial resolution. Many aspects of physical optics were ignored, and for them the reader is referred to reviews by Snyder (1979), Kunze (1979) and Land (1981) on invertebrates and Westheimer (1965, 1979) on humans. Though the fundamental principles underlying the optics of most visual systems are known, some of their details still remain to be answered. For example, what paths do incident light rays take through a receptor? Do they traverse the entire length of the outer segment and the rhabdoms? In the absence of signal summation and screening-pigment migration, how does the "effective" diameter of a receptor compare with the anatomical diameter of the pigment-containing organelle? The first two questions will be further considered in Section 5.2.

In as much as image-formation in cephalopods is the same as in vertebrates, spatial resolution among organisms will be exemplified next with illustrations from only vertebrate and compound eyes.

2.4.1 Vertebrate eye

The resolving power of the human eye has been extensively studied for over a century. Humans have been favored experimental subjects in the field of vision because they can readily and reliably

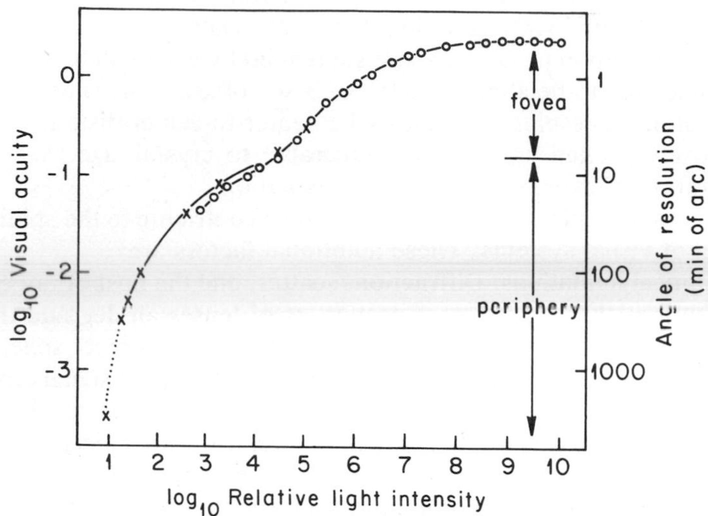

Figure 2.5. Visual acuity of the freely moving human eye as a function of light intensity, using Landolt's C as a visual target. Visual acuity, which is defined in text, is plotted on the left. The corresponding minimum resolvable angle is plotted on the right. The break in the smooth curve corresponds to the transition from peripheral to foveal vision. Data are from: ×, Pirenne et al. (1957) and ○, Shlaer (1937). Nowadays, sinusoidally varying spatial gratings are used as visual targets in more rigorous tests of acuity. (After Pirenne, 1962.)

indicate their visual experience. The subfield of psychology that quantitatively correlates the physical properties of a stimulus with the evoked human response is known as *psychophysics*. The results of a psychophysical experiment on visual resolution are illustrated in Figure 2.5. In this study subjects were asked to view a black letter C (called Landolt's C) against a white background and were asked whether they could discern the gap in the C. The subjects could freely move their heads, so they viewed the target with their most sensitive retinal regions. At any given background intensity, the letter's dimension was proportionately increased or decreased till its gap could be just resolved; that is, C was just barely distinguished from O. The angle subtended by the gap was then the minimum resolvable angle. By convention, *visual acuity* is defined as the reciprocal of the minimum resolvable angle expressed in minutes of arc.

The experimental subjects in Figure 2.5 used the foveal region of the retina when the intensity of the white background was increased. As shown, foveal acuity eventually achieved an angular resolution of 30 sec of arc, an angle subtended by a 0.15-mm-large object held at arms' length. This indeed is what would be predicted from foveal cone density using Equation (2.1) (with a 2.8-μm inter-receptor distance and a 17-mm focal length). The highest acuities yet verified for vertebrates belong to the birds of prey. The resolving power of the eagle is two to three times greater than that of the human (Shlaer, 1972).

As seen in the break of the curve in Figure 2.5, visual acuity in the peripheral retina corresponds, at best, to about 10 min of arc. This is a reflection of rod vision because rods are the predominant receptors in the peripheral retina. Separate experiments with subjects lacking cone function (rod monochromats) have confirmed this conclusion; the minimum resolvable angle with rod vision is actually about 6 min of arc (König, 1897; Hecht et al., 1948). Such an angle includes about 100 rods on the retinal surface and is an indication that the human visual system pools rod responses.

2.4.2 Compound eye

Spatial resolution in the compound eye is complicated by the fact that eyes with fused and unfused rhabdoms require separate consideration. For the sake of simplicity, the following discussion will be limited to eyes with fused rhabdoms, which were illustrated in Figure 2.2. In such eyes, the acceptance angle of every receptor within an individual ommatidium overlaps so much that all cells can be considered to share the same acceptance angle. As a result, the inter-receptor angle, which ultimately determines resolution, is replaced by the *interommatidial angle*. The smaller the interommatidial angle, that is, the flatter the eye's surface, the more ommatidia point in a given direction and, hence, the greater the resolution. The acceptance angle of individual ommatidia can reduce this optical resolution whenever it markedly exceeds the interommatidial angle. Because of screening-pigment migration, acceptance angles are a function of ambient light intensity.

Just as in vertebrates, resolution varies across the visual field of a compound eye. Figure 2.6 illustrates both the interommatidial and acceptance angles along one facet row in the apposition eye of the praying mantis. Note that the two angles are nearly the same. The best resolution is achieved in front of the animal, where the observed interommatidial angles are about 40 min of arc. In terms of resolution, this region is analogous to the vertebrate fovea and is marked as such

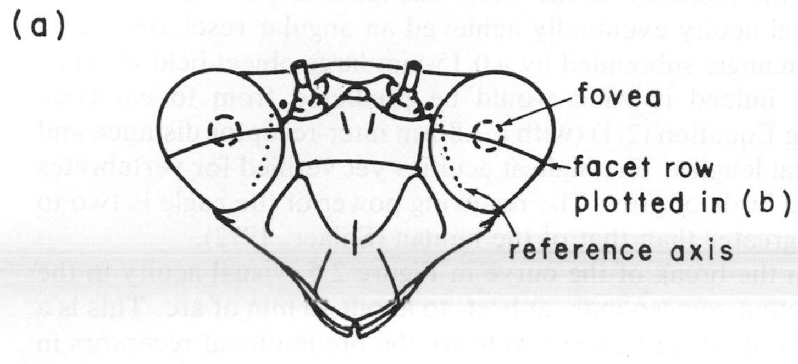

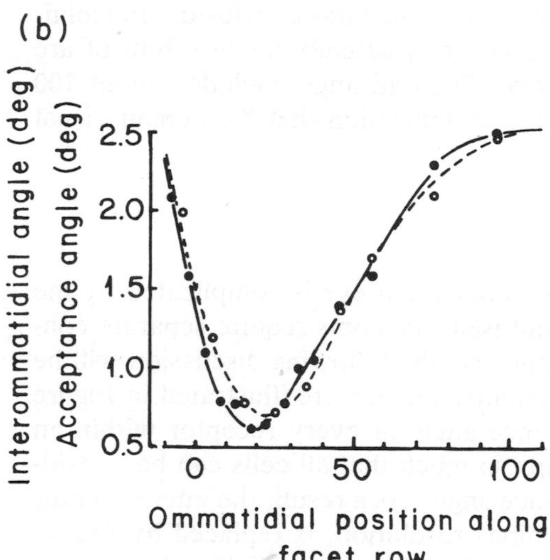

Figure 2.6. Acceptance and interommatidial angles for the compound eye of the praying mantis: (*a*) Frontal view of the mantis head, showing one of the reference axes used for identifying individual facets across the surface of the eye. Because the eyes are hemispheric, only about half of their surface is visible from a frontal vantage point. Fovea indicates the region with the highest resolution. (*b*) Distribution of interommatidial angles (●) and ommatidial acceptance angles (○) along a specific facet row. The acceptance angles were obtained under light-adapted conditions (see Chapter 8). (After Rossel, 1979.)

in Figure 2.6*a*. The highest acuity yet observed for a compound eye belongs to the dragonfly, whose interommatidial angle at its ''fovea'' is 15 min of arc (Sherk, 1978). Thus, the optimum resolving power of a compound eye is about 100 fold less than that of a vertebrate eye.

2.5 Summary

Although eye structures vary greatly among phyla and classes and sometimes even between the orders of a given class, they share an underlying organizational basis that is dictated by the need for image formation. This need dictates certain characteristic features of ocular organization. Consequently, complex eyes typically contain both a refractile apparatus capable of good image formation and a large number of densely packed photoreceptors in the focal plane.

3 Photoreceptor structure

The general anatomical features of eyes, which were discussed in the previous chapter, set the stage for a more detailed consideration of photoreceptor structure. Just as the cellular organization of an eye affects its overall optical performance, so does the subcellular and microscopic organization of a photoreceptor affect its functional properties. The structure of a photoreceptor is constrained by underlying cellular processes and, as will be discussed in Chapter 11, reveals considerable information about its molecular mechanism of photoreceptor excitation. This chapter on photoreceptor structure, consequently, will provide the reader with a basic introduction to photoreceptor physiology.

3.1 General characteristics

The morphological feature that distinguishes photoreceptors from other visual neurons is their tremendous proliferation of specialized membranes. To provide a reasonable photosensitivity, photoreceptors require a large number of visual pigment molecules, and because these molecules are integral membrane proteins, the membranes containing them must possess a large surface area. As a rule, photoreceptors contain in excess of one million rhodopsin molecules. Take the human rod as an example. It is capable of absorbing 1 photon sec^{-1} when the incident intensity of a continuous source of green light is about 4.6×10^7 photons sec^{-1}-cm^{-2} (Wald et al., 1963), about the brightness of the full moon. (The visual system's absolute threshold (see Table 1.2) is about four orders of magnitude lower than this intensity, mainly because the retina pools the signals from many rods.) The absorption cross section of a single rhodopsin molecule is about 2 $Å^2$, or 2×10^{-16} cm^2 (see Section 4.6). If the human rod contained only a single rhodopsin, an incident intensity of 4.6×10^7 photons sec^{-1}-cm^{-2} would lead to the absorption of only 9.2×10^{-9} photons sec^{-1}, or about 1 photon yr^{-1}. To reach a sufficiently high probability of catching at least 1 photon sec^{-1}, the human rod needs at least 10^8 rhodopsin molecules. This, in fact, is within an order of magnitude of the actual number present. Though this calculation was performed for a human rod, similar considerations apply for all photoreceptors. Such calculations illustrate that the absolute sensitivity of a receptor ultimately depends on the number of rhodopsin molecules it contains. The proliferation of pigmented membranes, which contain the large number of rhodopsin molecules, is the most characteristic feature of photoreceptors.

Because of their large surface area, pigmented membranes are generally folded to occupy a relatively compact volume. Interestingly, in all receptors known to date, this membrane formation, with its resulting structure, is based on one of two possible schemes: ciliary and rhabdomeric. The former, which is found in the eyes of protists, coelenterates, bryozoans, arrowworms, and chordates, refers to the infolding of nonmotile cilia's plasma membranes. Their pigmented membranes are flattened lamellae. For rhabdomeric receptors, cilia are absent; their pigmented membranes, which are also foldings of the plasma membrane, form cylindrical microvilli. Rhabdomeric receptors are observed in arthropods, annelids, mollusks, and flatworms. These two receptor types may represent divergent lines of evolutionary development (Eakin, 1963). Their separation, however, is not absolute because several organisms are known to contain both cell types, the best-known example being scallops (genus *Pecten*) (e.g., Barber et al., 1967).

3.2 Vertebrate photoreceptors

Vertebrate photoreceptors are ciliated cells, which were initially classified by early nineteenth-century biologists as either *rods* or *cones* on the basis of their appearance in the light microscope. These terms were originally coined to describe the geometrical shape of the distal tips of the receptors. Figure 3.1 demonstrates these features for the bullfrog (*Rana catesbeiana*) retina. Note the way the cones taper from their wide inner segments to the tip of their outer segments. Cones are not always dwarfed by rods, as seen here in the frog; they are the more massive and prominent cells in primate and fish retinas.

Because over the years many contrasting features were found between rods and cones, these receptors were once considered to be well-defined, distinct cell types. It is now realized that few, if any, of their morphological features are unique to either one of them. For example, foveal cones do not taper; rather, they are cylindrical and, on the basis of their shape, are indistinguishable from rods. Many other

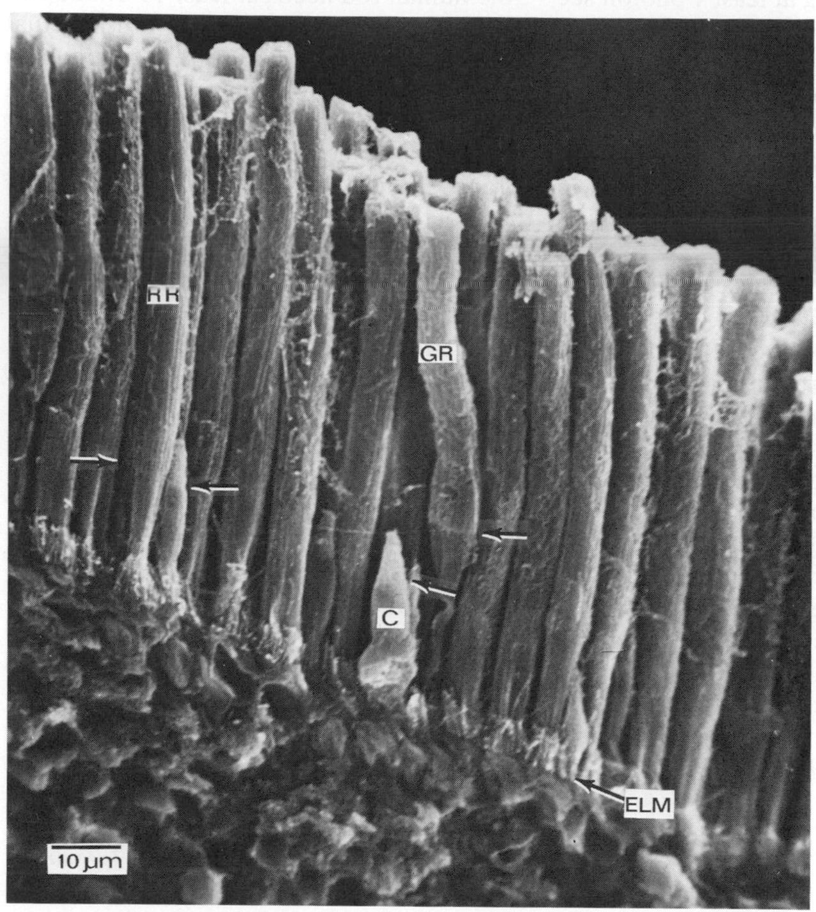

Figure 3.1. Scanning electron micrograph of the bullfrog (*Rana catesbeiana*) retina, showing the characteristic features of the receptors distal to the external limiting membrane (ELM). The pigment epithelium was removed to expose the photoreceptors, leaving behind the fine polysaccharide matrix, which appears as a gossamer material between the outer segments within the subretinal space. All the large cells are rods, whose two types, red rods (RR) and green rods (GR), can be seen here. The shorter and smaller photoreceptors are cones (C). Unlabeled arrows indicate the location of the ciliary bridge that joins the outer segment to the inner segment. (Courtesy of Steven L. Goodman.)

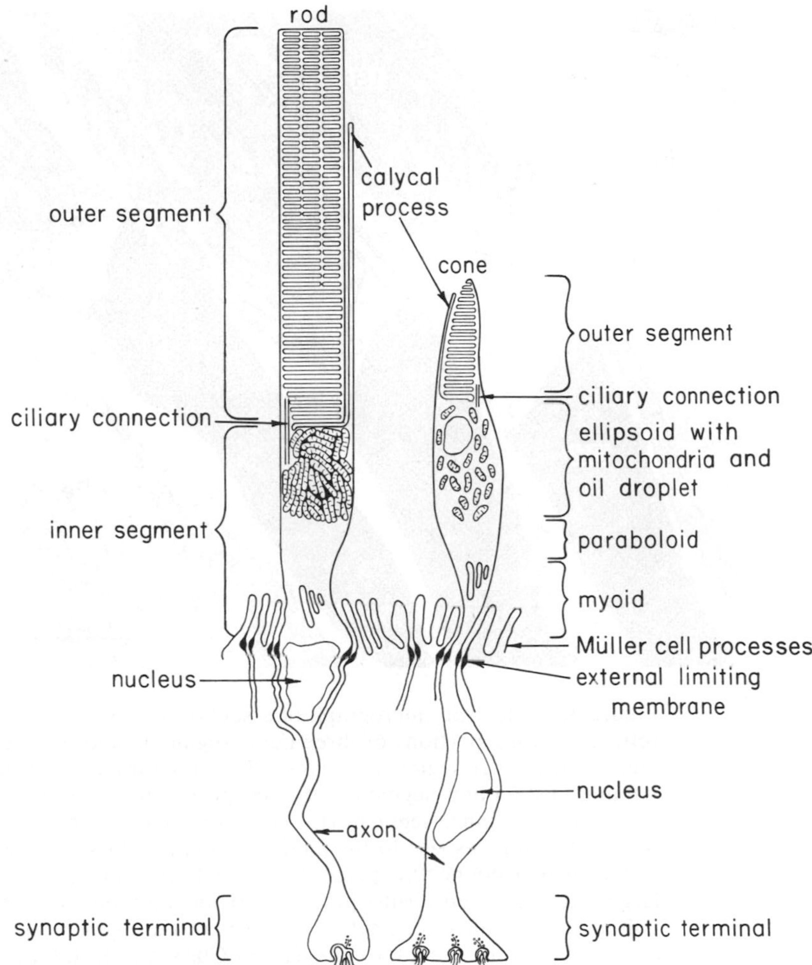

Figure 3.2. Schematic representation of "typical" rods and cones, showing major subcellular structures. See text for a full description. (After Nilsson, 1964.)

morphological hybrids exist, and some of these have been cited by Walls (1942) in the formulation of his theory for vertebrate photoreceptor evolution. Though it is still useful to talk about "typical" rods and cones, their classification can no longer be based on morphology alone. Functional properties such as photosensitivity and spatial and temporal resolution must also be considered.

The schematic drawing in Figure 3.2 demonstrates the major mor-

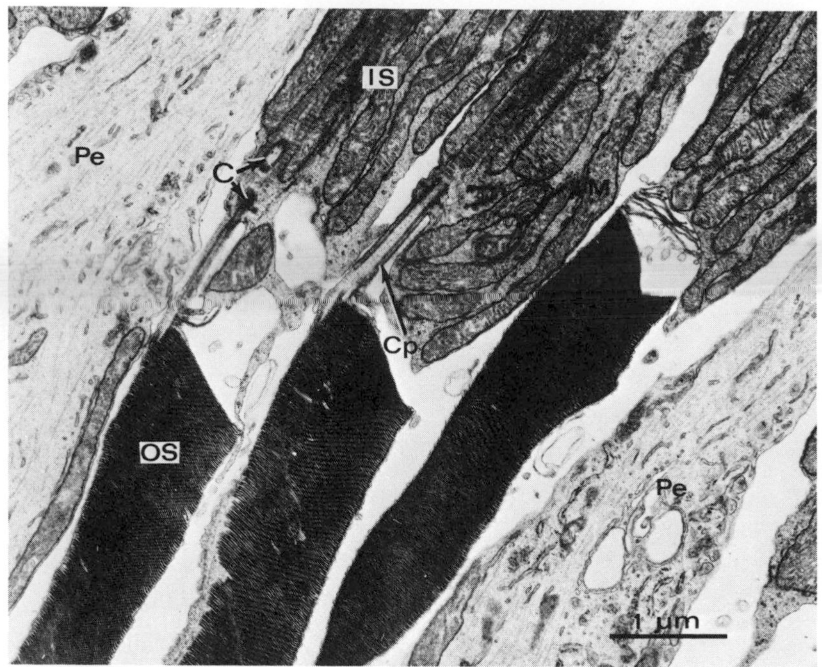

Figure 3.3. Electron micrograph of a section through a guinea pig retina, showing portions of three outer segments and their attachment to the inner segments. Disks, which take up most of the volume of the outer segment (OS), are perpendicular to the cell's long axis. The inner segment (IS) contains a pair of centrioles (C), one of which gives rise to the modified cilium, which is composed of the smaller connecting piece (Cp), or ciliary bridge, and the larger outer segment. Mitochrondria (M) occupy most of the volume of the inner segments. Processes of the pigment epithelium (Pe) ensheath the receptor cells. (From Clark and Branton, 1968.)

phological features of "typical" rods and cones. The compartmentalization of their subcellular organelles evident in this figure is characteristic of vertebrate receptors. The reader should refer to this figure for the subsequent discussion of specific cellular regions.

3.2.1 The outer segment

The *outer segment* is the site of phototransduction, where conversion of light energy into an electrical signal occurs. Its pigmented membranes, or *disks,* are infoldings of the plasma membrane

Table 3.1. *Common parameters for a frog rod outer segment with dimensions of 50* μm *(length)* $\times$ *6* μm *(diameter)*

Parameter	Value
Volumes	
Total volume per outer segment	1.4 pl
Extradiskal volume per outer segment	0.7 pl
Internal aqueous volume per single disk[a]	60 al[b]
Surfaces	
Number of disks per outer segment	1700
Surface area per disk	56 μm^2
Plasma membrane area per outer segment (neglecting basal disk invaginations)	1000 μm^2
Ratio of total disk area to plasma membrane area	94
Rhodopsin values	
Rhodopsin molecules per outer segment[c]	2.5×10^9
Rhodopsin molecules per disk	1.5×10^6
Rhodopsin areal density	2.7×10^4 molecules/μm^2
Rhodopsins per retina[d]	10 nmoles
Photoreceptors	
Rod cells per retina[d]	2×10^6

[a] With disk membranes 20 Å apart.
[b] Prefix atto (a) refers to the multiplier 10^{-18}.
[c] With overall rhodopsin concentration being 3 mM.
[d] Varies with the size of the retina.

and are oriented perpendicular to the long axis of the outer segment (Figure 3.3). Besides disks, microtubules are the only other structures that can be observed with an electron microscope in this part of the cell.

Both X-ray diffraction measurements on excised retinas (Blaurock and Wilkins, 1969) and freeze-fracture studies (Korenbrot et al., 1973) indicate that the center-to-center distance between adjacent disks has a constant value of about 300 Å and remains about the same in most rods and cones. Given this spacing, the number of disks within an outer segment can be easily calculated once its length is known. Table 3.1 lists this and other calculated parameters for a typical frog rod outer segment. Because the entire thickness of a disk is half of the repeat distance, the cytoplasmic volume is only 50% of the outer segment volume. The internal membrane surfaces of a disk are separated by a 20

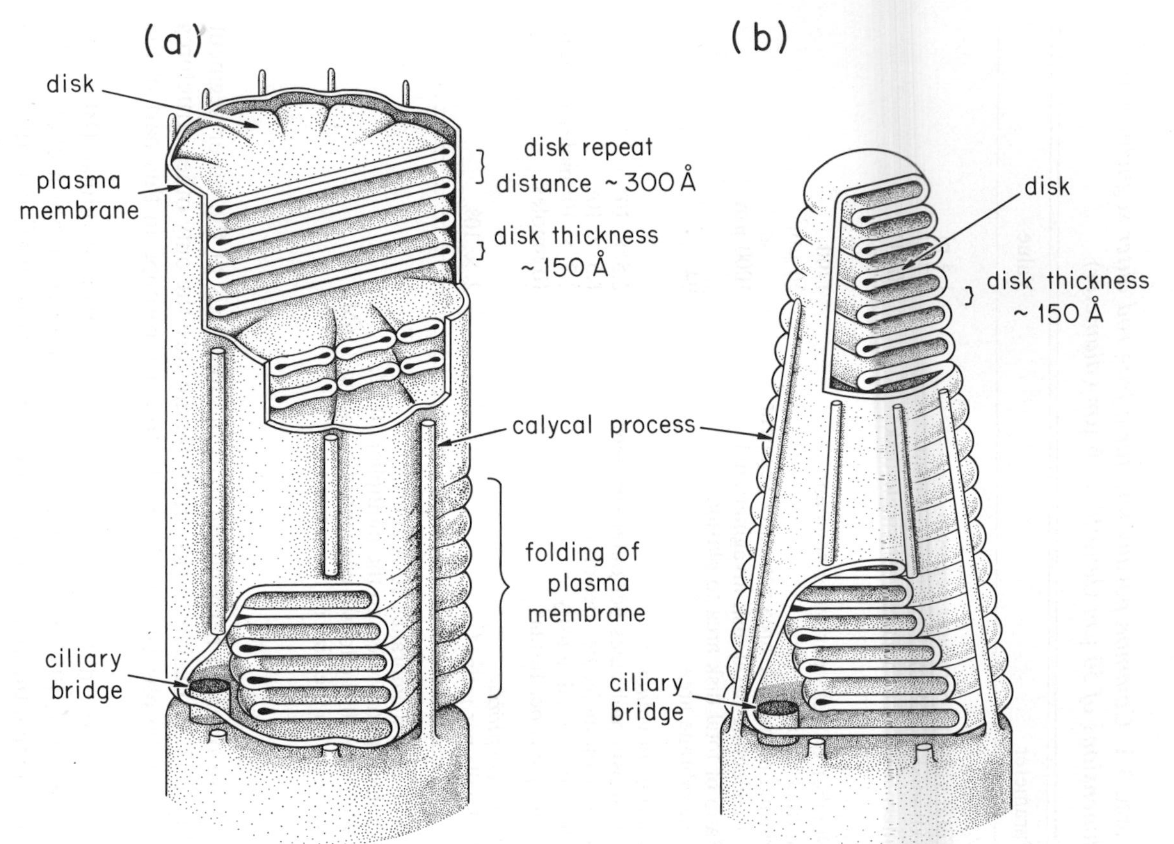
(a)
disk
plasma membrane
disk repeat distance ~ 300 Å
disk thickness ~ 150 Å
calycal process
folding of plasma membrane
ciliary bridge
(b)
disk
disk thickness ~ 150 Å
ciliary bridge

± 5-Å-wide aqueous space (Chabre and Cavaggioni, 1975), which is maintained over the entire extent of the disk.

Microspectrophotometry on individual cells and spectral measurements on purified disks have proven that the visual pigment is localized to the outer segment region of the cell. Though the pigment is embedded within both disk and plasma membranes (Jan and Revel, 1974; Rüppel and Hagins, 1973), over 90% of it resides in the disks, whose surface area is much larger (Table 3.1). Rhodopsin concentration within the outer segment is 3 to 3.5 mM in several amphibian rods (Harosi, 1975; Liebman, 1975) and may well be the same for most other cells (Harosi, 1976). Using this concentration value, it can be calculated that typical frog rods contain about 3×10^9 rhodopsin molecules (see Table 3.1).

Disk topology characteristically differs between rods and cones (Figure 3.4). The disks of "typical" cones are continuous with the plasma membrane, and thus their internal space is filled with an extracellular solution. In rods, however, aside from a few basal disks nearest the ciliary junction, all disks are pinched off from the plasma membrane, with each disk forming a closed, intracellular vesicle. The evidence for this characteristic rod property, which has important implications for the mechanism of transduction, is firmly based on electron microscopy (Cohen, 1972) and on electrophysiological observations (Murakami and Pak, 1970; Penn and Hagins, 1972). Although the rod disks are pinched off the plasma membrane, they are not free floating, as is often erroneously stated. Their rims are connected to the plasma membrane by as yet unidentified structures. The existence of these connections is inferred because hypotonic shocks (equivalent to pressure differentials of several atmospheres) are ineffective in disrupting the association between disk rims and the plasma membrane (Cohen, 1971; Szuts, 1975). As Figures 3.2 and 3.4 illustrate, parallel to and in close proximity with each outer segment are long, slender (about 100 nm

Figure 3.4. Schematic representation of the membrane topology of rod and cone outer segments. The relationship of the calycal processes with the outer segments is shown, but the details of the inner segment and connecting cilium are omitted. In all receptors, disks are formed by the infolding of the plasma membrane at the basal end of the outer segment. (*a*) In rods, the disks eventually pinch off the cell membrane and form isolated vesicles. Only the most basal 10–20 disks retain their continuity with the plasma membrane. (*b*) In cones, all the disks maintain their attachment to the membrane. As shown here for frog cones, the region of attachment is extensive for each disk and is in register between adjacent neighbors. (After Young, 1970.)

diameter), fingerlike structures called *calycal processes* (Cohen, 1972). They are outgrowths of the inner segments and their physiological function remains unclear.

3.2.2 The inner segment

The aforementioned outer segments are modified nonmotile cilia that are outgrowths of the *inner segments*. A slender ciliary bridge (Figure 3.3) connects the inner and outer regions of the receptor. The inner segment consists of three regions: ellipsoid, paraboloid, and myoid (see Figure 3.2). The *ellipsoid* is characterized by a very dense accumulation of mitochondria, which supply the cell's metabolic energy. In some birds, amphibians, and reptiles, cone ellipsoids may also contain large oil droplets, which are often brilliantly colored. Because they are pigmented and because light must pass through them before being absorbed by the rhodopsin, they, in essence, act like color filters, substantially altering the spectral sensitivity of photoreceptors. Proximal to the ellipsoid is the *paraboloid,* which contains intracellular vacuoles and presumptive glycogen granules. The *myoid* is characterized by the organelles normally associated with protein synthesis: free ribosomes, rough endoplasmic reticulum, and Golgi apparatus. It is also rich in contractile proteins, which are responsible for the photomechanical movements observed in some species. The ability to change its shape is the source of its name; myoid means musclelike. Photomechanical responses, which are regulated by the receptor's state of adaptation, will be extensively discussed in Chapter 8.

3.2.3 The nucleus and the synaptic terminal

Moving proximally along the cell, the next region to be encountered is the cell body. It is almost always located proximal to the *external limiting membrane,* which is not a true membrane but rather a region of tight junctions between receptors and Müller cells. The origin of its name is attributed to the fact that the junctions readily accumulate stain and so appear as a dense line when retinal sections are observed with the low resolution of the light microscope. A long, narrow *axon* (also called fiber), with a diameter of about 1 μm, connects the nuclear region with the synaptic terminal.

The *synaptic terminal,* which is the site of information transfer to the higher-order retinal neurons, is just as important a cellular region as the outer segment. Photoreceptors contact horizontal and bipolar cells (see Figure 2.1*b*) via chemical synapses and employ both electrical and

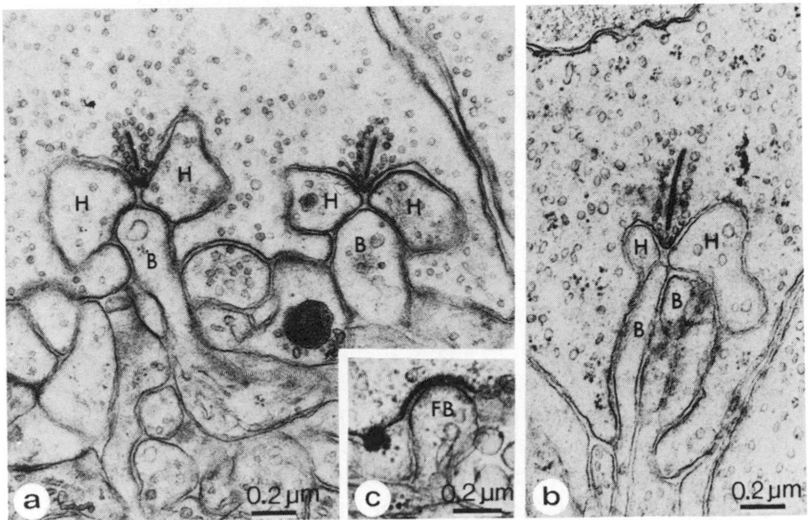

Figure 3.5. High-power electron micrographs of receptor synapses. (*a*) In cone terminals, each ribbon synapse makes contact with three postsynaptic processes. (*b*) In rod terminals, four or more processes are observed per ribbon. In both rods and cones, the processes that lie laterally deeper in the invaginations are horizontal cell processes (H); the central elements are bipolar cell dendrites (B). (*c;* center) A superficial contact of a flat bipolar (FB) on a cone terminal. (From Dowling, 1970.)

chemical synapses to interact with each other. Although chemical synapses are confined to the synaptic terminal, the location of interreceptor gap junctions, which are the presumptive sites of electrical coupling, may be variable. In toad rods, for example, these gap junctions are found near the fiber baskets at the inner segment level (Gold and Dowling, 1979). On the basis of its size and shape, the synaptic terminal is called *pedicle* in cones and *spherule* in rods. Rod spherules are smaller than pedicles and generally contain only a single deep invagination into which the dendrites of the second-order neurons insert. By contrast, cone pedicles have a flattened base that is invaded with numerous, but shallow, invaginations.

Because of its characteristic feature, the typical chemical synapse of a photoreceptor is known as a *ribbon synapse* (Figure 3.5). Though it shares many similarities with a conventional synapse, its distinguishing feature is a densely staining synaptic ribbon, which is about 300 Å thick in cross section, about 0.5 μm wide, and 1 μm long (Gray and Pease,

1971). Ribbon synapses are not unique to photoreceptors. They can also be found in some of the bipolar cells of the vertebrate retina. Moreover, structures similar to the synaptic ribbon have been reported in a few arthropod photoreceptors (Trujillo-Cenoz, 1965) and in the hair cells of the cochlea (Smith and Sjöstrand, 1961). Though most of the synaptic contacts between photoreceptors and higher-order neurons occur at ribbon synapses, less prominent contacts can also be observed between them (Figure 3.5*c*).

Compartmentalization in vertebrate receptors extends beyond gross morphology into some interesting aspects of molecular organization. The physiology of vertebrate receptors will be discussed in some detail subsequently. It is sufficient to say at this point that in the dark an ionic current can be measured in the subretinal space surrounding the receptors. This current leaves the cell at the inner segment, flows distally, and enters the outer segment. The current is detectable only because its source and sink are compartmentalized to different regions of the cell; that is, the associated membrane molecules (ionic pumps and channels) are nonuniformly distributed. The nervous system is replete with many examples of neurons whose membrane properties are similarly segregated to specific regions.

3.3 Invertebrate photoreceptors

The pigmented membranes of invertebrates are typically microvillar in nature. *Microvilli* are cylindrical foldings of the plasma membrane that are variable in dimension, whether the comparison is made among species or among the villi of the very same cell. Their axial lengths can range between 1 and 10 μm, and their diameters, between 0.05 and 0.1 μm. In compound eyes, where the long axes of the microvilli are perpendicular to the visual axis, the microvilli usually pack into a highly regular hexagonal array (Figure 3.8). Microspectrophotometric measurements have established that the microvilli are the sites where the visual pigments are imbedded in the membranes (Langer and Thorell, 1966; Goldsmith et al., 1968). Invertebrate visual pigments are also called rhodopsins because they share many of the properties of their vertebrate analogs (see Chapter 4).

Though the morphological variety among invertebrate eyes is greater than among vertebrates, the similarity of their receptors outweighs the need for a genus-by-genus survey of receptor ultrastructure. Because a preponderance of our knowledge about invertebrates was derived from electrophysiological and ultrastructural studies performed on *Limulus*, we shall focus on the receptors of this organism for our subsequent discussion.

Table 3.2. *Common parameters for* Limulus *photoreceptors*

Parameter	Ventral eye[a]	Lateral compound eye[b]
Microvilli		
Axial length	~1 μm[c]	1–2.5 μm
Diameter	0.07 μm[c]	0.1 μm
Microvilli per receptor	2×10^5	5×10^5
Surfaces		
Microvilli membrane per receptor	3×10^4 μm²	3×10^5 μm²
Fraction of plasma membrane occupied by microvilli	0.9	unavailable
Volumes		
Internal volume of a microvillus	4 al	13 al
Total volume per cell body	0.4 nl[d]	0.1 nl[e]
Rhodopsin		
Molecules of rhodopsin per receptor	10^9	10^{10}
Photoreceptors		
Receptors per ommatidium	–	12[f]
Receptors per eye	300[g]	8000[g]

[a] Based on data from Lisman and Bering, 1977.
[b] Based on data from Fahrenbach, 1969.
[c] From Clark et al., 1969.
[d] For a prolate cell with dimensions given in Figure 3.6*b*.
[e] The aggregate of ommatidial receptors normally occupies a prolate-shaped volume, with a 300-μm major axis and 200-μm minor axis (Figure 2.2 *a*). To obtain the volume of a single cell body, the aggregate's volume was divided by the average number of receptors.
[f] This is an average, as the number varies from 4 to 20.
[g] From Fahrenbach, 1975.

3.3.1 Typical photoreceptor of a simple eye

A light micrograph and a schematic drawing of a single *Limulus* ventral photoreceptor are shown in Figure 3.6. Resembling the receptors of the most rudimentary simple eyes, its rhabdomeres are randomly distributed along the highly convoluted surface of its cell body. The ovoid soma attains dimensions that are about 200 μm in length and 60 μm in width. Using early receptor potential measurements (see Chapter 6), Lisman and Bering (1977) estimate the visual pigment content to be about 10^9 rhodopsin molecules per cell. Given rhodopsin's normal areal density, the number of microvilli per cell is then about 2×10^5 (see Table 3.2). Within the cell body, most of the

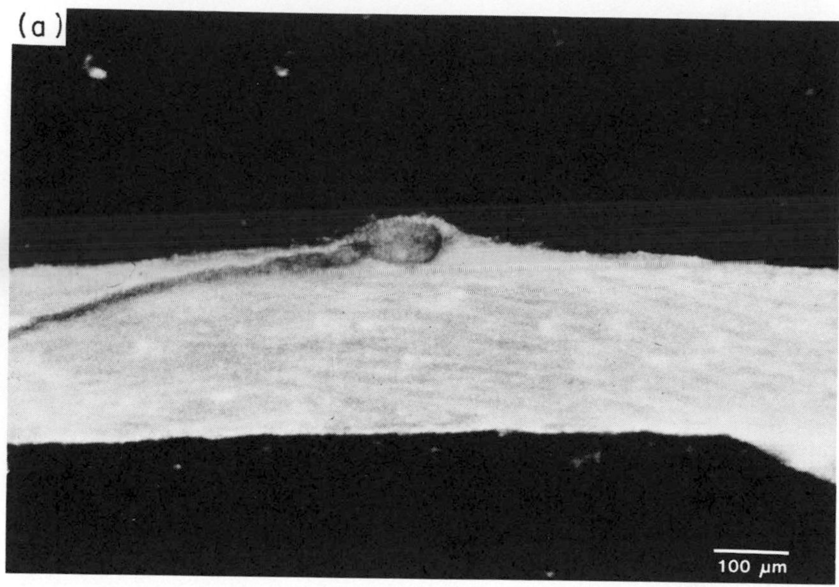

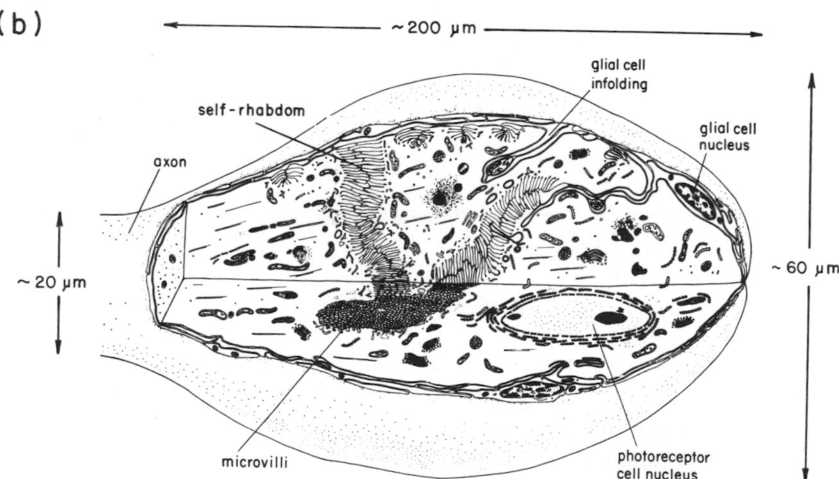

Figure 3.6. Photoreceptors from the ventral eye of *Limulus*. (*a*) Light micrograph of a single receptor filled with horseradish peroxidase reaction products. (*b*) Schematic representation of a single receptor with a few of its glial cells. A segment of the cell body was removed to show the approximate relationships of the intracellular organelles. (After Clark et al., 1969.)

microvilli fold upon each other, forming tip-to-tip junctions – arrangements that have been called *self-rhabdoms* (Jones et al., 1971). Although membrane cisternae are often seen near the rhabdomeres, no major structures such as the palisade of the lateral compound eye are discerned within the soma.

Fahrenbach (1975) has noted that the distribution of glial cells in the visual system of *Limulus* is inversely related to the abundance of pigmented supporting cells. No pigment cells are associated with ventral eye photoreceptors and their absence greatly simplifies quantification of light stimuli. However, the receptors are smothered with light-transparent glial cells, only a few of which are shown in Figure 3.6*b*. These glial cells, which cover the entire surface of the receptor, may be as many as ten layers thick, and they routinely send processes deep into the receptor soma. In spite of these invaginations, which may also contain efferent axons, no high-resistance pathway occurs between the extracellular space of deep rhabdomeres and the outside (Brown et al., 1979). The unrestricted passage of extracellular ions through the glial layers greatly facilitates the interpretation of electrophysiological studies.

3.3.2 *Typical photoreceptor of a compound eye*

The gross morphology of a *Limulus* ommatidium was shown in Figure 2.2. A more detailed schematic drawing of the receptors appears in Figure 3.7. Each retinular cell contains about 4×10^5 microvilli, all aligned perpendicular to the ommatidial axis (Figure 3.8). Given the size of the microvilli (Figure 3.8) and the usual density of rhodopsin in membranes, it can be calculated that there are about 10^{10} rhodopsins per retinular cell (see Table 3.2). The eccentric cell dendrite, which is also covered with microvilli, most likely does not contain rhodopsin because the cell itself appears to be insensitive to light (Smith and Baumann, 1969). The microvilli of the eccentric cell form junctions with all the surrounding retinular cells, presumably ensuring strong electrical coupling between them. The rhabdoms are the only sites where retinular cells contact each other – their nonvillous plasma membranes are separated by pigment cells. The cytoplasm adjacent to the microvilli (that is, the space between the rhabdomeric spokes) is occupied by an extensive system of membraneous cisterns called a *palisade* (Figure 3.8). Its exact function is as yet unknown, although it is likely to be directly involved in the membrane turnover, as recently described by Chamberlain and Barlow (1978). Thus it is not surprising that the structure of the palisade varies with the state of light adaptation.

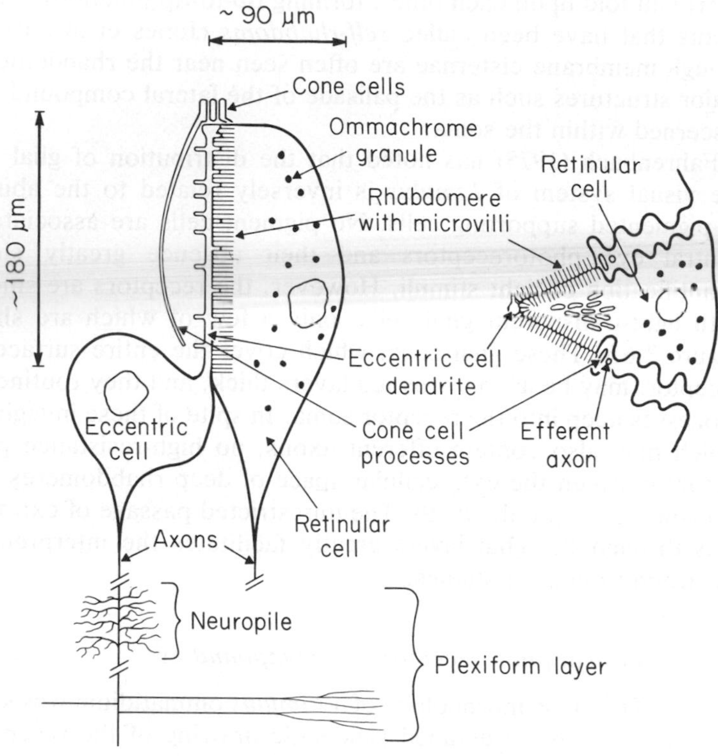

Figure 3.7. Schematic drawing of a single retinular cell from the compound eye of *Limulus*. Pigment cells, which completely surround the retinular cell away from the microvilli, are not shown. See text for a full description.

Apart from their rhabdomeres and palisades, *Limulus* retinular cells show little structural compartmentalization. Their soma is prominently filled with large amounts of endoplasmic reticulum, ribosomes, and membrane-bound pigment granules known as *ommochromes*. The location of these granules with respect to the rhabdom is related to light adaptation and will be discussed in Chapter 8. On leaving the ommatidia, the eccentric and retinular cell axons form the lateral optic tract, which weaves an indirect 5-cm-long pathway to the brain. Apparently, all eccentric and retinular cells synapse directly onto the cells of the first optic ganglion, which is known as the *lamina*. Because action potentials are generated by eccentric cells but not by retinular cells, the importance of the retinular cell axons is not yet known; their visual function has not been adequately investigated. An important property

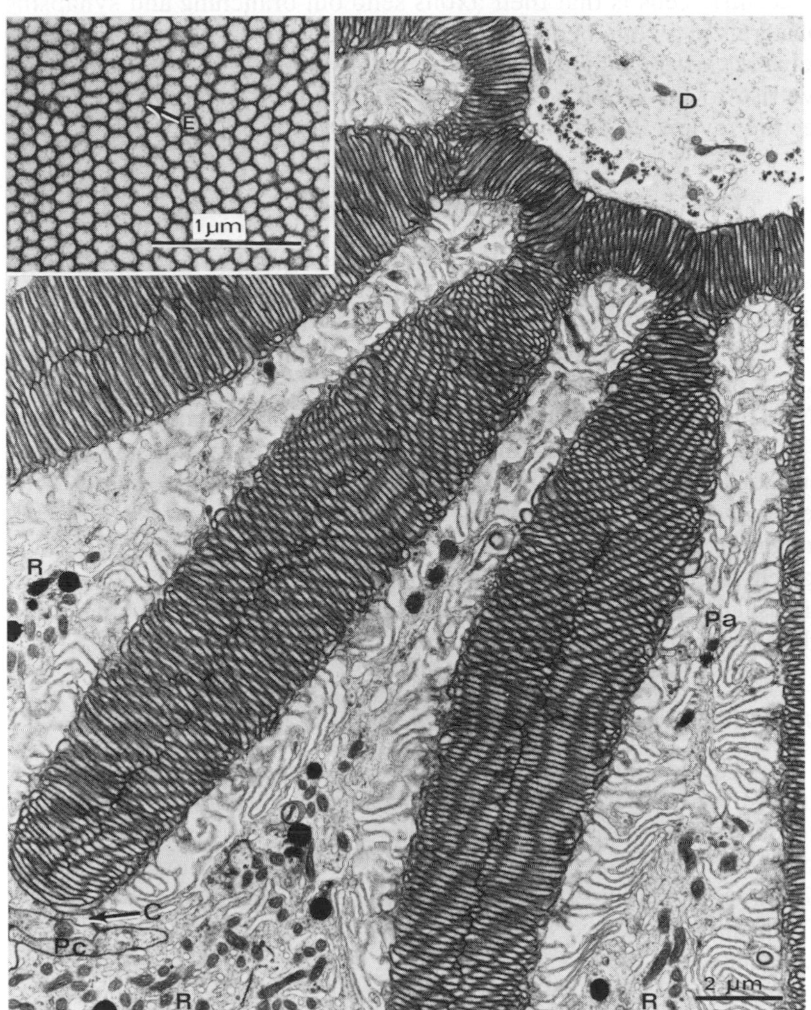

Figure 3.8. Electron micrographs of retinular cells from a *Limulus* compound eye, showing a section perpendicular to the ommatidial axis through the eccentric cell dendrite (D) and the rhabdomeres of four retinular cells. Note how the microvilli lie within the plane of the section. The palisade (Pa) is seen in its fully formed, dark-adapted condition. Within the broad partition separating adjacent retinular cells (R), cone cell processes (C) and the pigment cells (Pc) can be observed. (From Fahrenbach, 1969.) Inset: Cross section through the rhabdomeric microvilli, which are packed into a loose hexagonal array, with their closely apposed membranes forming tight junctions. Note the small extracellular space (E). (Courtesy of Wolf H. Fahrenbach.)

of eccentric cells is that their axons send out branching and synapsing collaterals in a zone beneath the ommatidial layer. They form a *plexus* (network) where inhibitory synapses between neighboring ommatidia give rise to the well-known *lateral inhibition* discovered by Hartline (see the review by Hartline and Ratliff, 1972).

3.4 Photoreceptor membrane turnover

Photoreceptors are not the static structures that the previous discussion would seem to imply. A general property of all biological cells is that they continuously rejuvenate themselves by an orderly process that destroys and resynthesizes their cellular components. Such a process is referred to as *turnover*. It has been said that only DNA, the genetic material, escapes turnover in somatic cells. Turnover studies in photoreceptors have been limited to the specific components of the pigmented membranes and synaptic vesicles, and even these have been thoroughly investigated in only a few species. Although the experimental evidence is still scant, it appears that visual pigment turnover is a general property of all photoreceptors. Not surprisingly, turnover rates in some animals are altered by changes in light and dark.

3.4.1 Turnover in vertebrates

The incontrovertible proof for rhodopsin turnover was first demonstrated in vertebrates by Young and co-workers (see the review by Young, 1976). For their studies, these investigators relied on autoradiographic techniques. In a typical experiment, radioactive amino acids are injected into the vitreous of the eye. The labeled amino acids diffuse throughout the extracellular space of the retinal tissue, are accumulated by the cells (among them the receptors), and eventually are incorporated into proteins. The location of the radioactively labeled proteins can be determined at any time if the retinas are fixed and sectioned, and the sections then placed in contact with a photographic emulsion. The β-rays emitted by the decaying atoms strike and expose the nearby silver halide crystals in the emulsion. Their pattern of exposure can be visualized after the film is developed by standard photographic techniques.

Figure 3.9 summarizes the results that Young and co-workers obtained when their autoradiography study was performed with frog rods. Following the accumulation of the labeled amino acids by the rods, the initial radioactivity is concentrated within the rod myoid, the primary region for protein synthesis (Figure 3.9*a*). The amino acids are

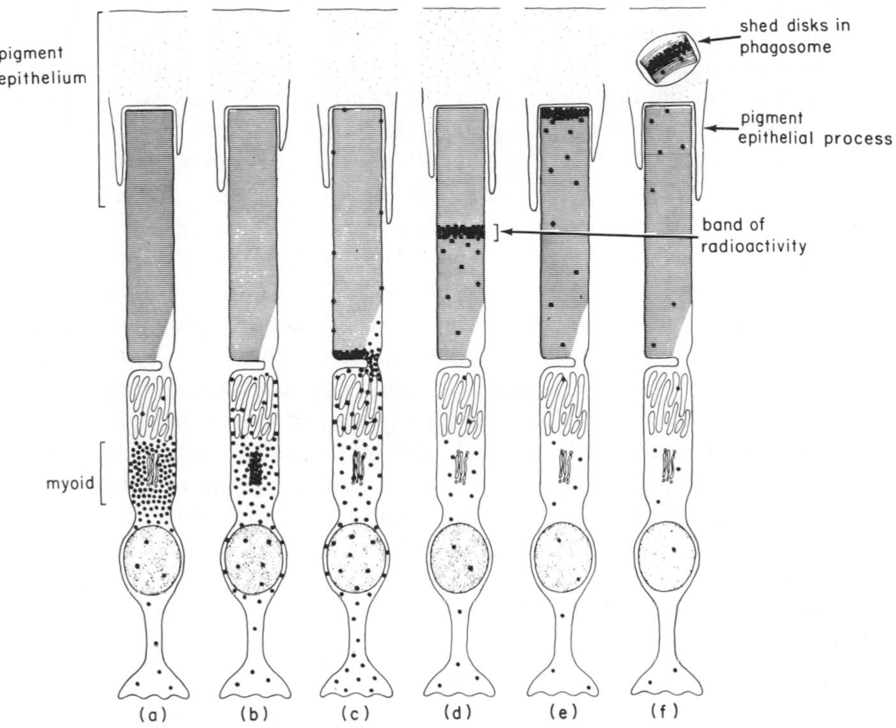

Figure 3.9. Diagram illustrating the renewal of protein in rods as it is revealed in autoradiograms after administration of radioactive amino acids. See text for full explanation. (After Young, 1976.)

incorporated into precursors of the visual pigment and of other cellular proteins. The protein molecules then travel throughout the cell, many of them migrating by way of the Golgi complex, where they are modified by the addition of carbohydrates (Figure 3.9*b*). Some of the labeled proteins, most of them being rhodopsins, subsequently migrate through the ciliary stalk to the outer segment, where they form a band of radioactivity (Figure 3.9*c*). With time, the band of labeled rhodopsins travels as a discrete unit toward the distal end of the rod (Figure 3.9*d*). The band of radioactivity stays unchanged in width throughout its axial movement. Depending on the species, about a month is required for the radioactive band to reach the rod tips (Figure 3.9*e*), where it is shed off to be phagocytized by the pigment epithelium (Figure 3.9*f*). Throughout this process, the length of the outer segment remains essentially unchanged. As Young and co-workers realized, a constant length implies a balance between disk synthesis and disk destruction. Rod disks are continuously synthesized by infoldings of the plasma membrane at the basal end of the outer segment. The rate of synthesis is obtained by dividing the number of disks per outer segment by the time interval needed for the band of radioactivity to migrate from the basal to the distal end of the outer segment. For frogs, this rate turns out to be 1700 disks per 60 days or 1.2 disks hr^{-1} (Young and Bok, 1969). Newly synthesized rhodopsin molecules, which are labeled in the autoradiographic experiments, are incorporated into disks only at the basal region. The rhodopsin molecules are then trapped in the disks when the latter pinch off from the plasma membrane. This explains why the band of radioactivity remains discrete on its axial journey – membrane-bound proteins, such as rhodopsin, cannot partition into the aqueous cytoplasm nor can they diffuse beyond the confines of their disk. The orderly process of disk synthesis and destruction appears to be extremely crucial to photoreceptor function. If the pigment epithelium is incapable of phagocytizing the shed disks, the rod cells eventually die off (Bok and Hall, 1971). Why the absence of disk destruction should signal receptor death is not yet known.

Rhodopsin turnover in cones most likely parallels that in rods even though no discrete band of radioactivity has ever been observed in cone outer segments. Its absence may well be due to the visual pigment's rapid diffusion (see Section 5.3.2). Because cone disks in frog are continuous with the plasma membrane, cone pigments can easily escape from the confines of a single disk. Similarity with rods moreover may also extend to disk shedding, which has been observed in both human and squirrel cones (Hogan et al., 1974; Anderson and Fisher, 1975). Thus it appears that the very same mechanism of disk synthesis and destruction operates in both rods and cones.

LaVail (1976*a*) discovered that in rats the animal's own circadian rhythm can cause a synchronized burst of disk shedding from rods. Though this burst of activity coincides with morning, with the onset of the circadian light period, light is not a direct stimulus. It is necessary only to keep the animal's biological clock entrained. A similar synchronous burst of disk shedding from the tips of lizard cones was observed by Young (1977), but here the burst of activity coincided with the onset of the circadian dark period. The identity of the circadian signal and its mechanism are unknown.

3.4.2 Turnover in invertebrates

Ultrastructural changes in association with light or darkness have been well documented for invertebrates (see the review by Eakin, 1972). The larval ocellus of the mosquito is one of the receptors in

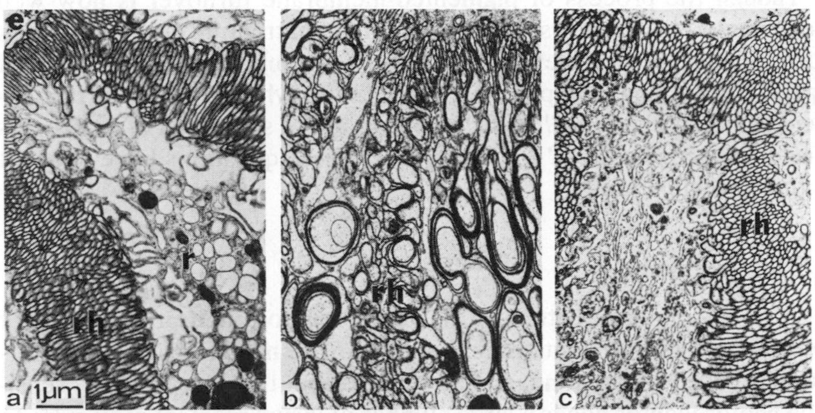

Figure 3.10. Electron micrographs showing the temporal sequence of rhabdom breakdown and reassembly in a *Limulus* compound eye. (*a*) Part of the rhabdom from a control animal that was not exposed to light. A retinular cell (r), one of the rhabdoms (rh) that it makes with the adjacent retinular cell, and the eccentric cell dendrite (e) are identified. (*b*) Rhabdom breakdown after 15 min of continuous exposure to sunlight. The microvillar array is disrupted and much of its membrane has been incorporated into lamellar bodies within the cytoplasm. (*c*) Reassembled rhabdom after 30 min of continuous exposure to sunlight. The microvillar array has been restored. Magnification identical for all three micrographs. (From Chamberlain and Barlow, 1979.)

which these ultrastructural changes suggest membrane turnover (White and Lord, 1975). The rhabdoms of these ocelli enlarge with darkness and diminish with light. Under persistent illumination, the rhabdoms attain a certain volume, which is inversely proportional to the logarithm of light's intensity. This observation indicates that under constant illumination a process of membrane assembly is balanced by disassembly. Whether the structures are synthesized de novo each time and then destroyed, as required for renewal, is not yet known.

A most dramatic observation has been reported by Chamberlain and Barlow (1979) for the compound eyes of *Limulus* (Figure 3.10). Provided that the efferent input from the brain to the eye remains functional, the microvilli of the retinular cells are synchronously destroyed with the first light of morning. The rhabdoms are subsequently rebuilt, with the entire process of destruction and renewal being completed within 30 min. It is clear that in *Limulus* this dramatic manifestation of membrane turnover is controlled by the animal's circadian rhythm.

Though the process of pigmented-membrane turnover is now well documented in receptors, it has raised many intriguing questions. Does turnover correct for inevitable errors in assembly or for the aging of specific membrane components? If the latter, which membrane component is most vulnerable? Is it rhodopsin, and if so, which of its properties does aging destroy? The answers to these questions have to await future investigations.

3.5 Summary

A common feature of all photoreceptors is a proliferation of cellular membranes containing rhodopsin. The need for such a proliferation is based on the fundamental requirement that a reasonably sensitive photoreceptor needs a large number of visual pigment molecules to ensure the absorption of a sufficient fraction of incident photons. Rhodopsin is a membrane protein, and therefore, to contain it in sufficient numbers, a large membrane area is required.

In terms of function, photoreceptors possess two important regions: the phototransduction site and the synaptic terminal. It is at the transduction site where the membrane proliferation occurs. Whether they are ciliary disks or rhabdomeric microvilli, the organization of these membranes shows a characteristic pattern that appears to be highly regular and even static. However, photoreceptors are highly dynamic structures whose rhodopsin-containing membranes undergo constant renewal.

4 General structure and spectral property of rhodopsin

The preceding two chapters introduced the reader to the general anatomy of eyes and photoreceptors. At this point, the discussion turns to the molecular processes of visual excitation that will be continued, with few digressions, for the rest of the book. The molecule to be considered first is rhodopsin, the visual pigment, which by absorbing a photon triggers the entire process of vision. Rhodopsin is so crucial to phototransduction that the next three chapters have been exclusively devoted to it, with this chapter considering its physical structure and spectral properties. The study of rhodopsin dates from the mid-1800s, and its historical highlights are worth reviewing before the discussion on the molecular structure of the molecule begins.

4.1 Historical background

The first recorded observations of retinal pigment colors are attributed to Krohn (1842) and to Müller (1851), who observed them in squid and frog retinas, respectively. Neither the origin nor the significance of these colors was recognized until 1876, when Boll discovered that the "red" color of frog rods is photosensitive and bleaches with illumination. Boll's discovery was the first proof that the rods and cones, which were by then known for many decades, were indeed photoreceptors. Boll correctly concluded that "this objective [color] change of the outer segments by light must undoubtedly be part of the act of seeing" (Boll, 1877). Within two months of Boll's announcement, Kühne proved that "visual red" is a true pigment, and he subsequently gave it the name by which we now refer to all visual pigments: *rhodopsin* (Greek for visual rose). (Sehpurpur, or "visual purple," was another term used coincidently by Kühne. Its use was unfortunate because to most observers, the rhodopsin of vertebrate rods is salmon pink in appearance without any hint of purple, as claimed by Kühne. This case illustrates the pitfalls of any pigment nomenclature based solely on subjective color appearance.) Kühne's subsequent studies of rhodopsin were very extensive, and after him not much more was learned about visual pigments for another half a century.

The next major advance occurred in 1933, when Wald discovered that rhodopsin contained a vitamin A derivative. Thus Wald provided the first evidence for the direct biological activity of vitamin A, although dietary night blindness was known since ancient Egypt and in 1925 was conclusively shown to be the initial symptom of vitamin A deficiency. Wald and his co-workers continued their study of visual pigments for several decades and provided many fundamental contributions to our current knowledge on the photochemistry of visual pigments.

4.2 Structure of visual pigments

As far as has been determined, all visual pigments in nature possess a similar structure. They are the reaction product of a large apoprotein known as *opsin* and a single prosthetic group called *retinal,* which are covalently bound to each other with a one-to-one stoichiometry.

4.2.1 The chromophore

Retinal is the light-absorbing part of the molecule and, as a result, is also called the visual pigment chromophore. As discovered by Morton and his co-workers (Ball et al., 1948), retinal is the aldehyde derivative of vitamin A. More specifically, it is a β-ionone ring linked to a five double-bonded polyene chain that terminates in an aldehyde group (Figure 4.1). When the aldehyde group, which is the most reactive part of the molecule, is reduced to an alcohol, the molecule is called *retinol,* or *vitamin A,* and when it is oxidized to a carboxylic acid, the product is called *retinoic acid.* Because retinal and all its derivatives are highly hydrophobic, they are insoluble in aqueous media.

The delocalized electrons within the conjugated bonds, along with the methyl groups, determine the conformation of the chromophore. Many stereoisomers, with either *cis* or *trans* conformation, exist about the five double bonds. Some of these are shown in Figure 4.2. These isomers retain their conformation in solution because the energy barriers separating them exceed the thermal energies available at normal temperatures. However, the barriers can be easily surmounted with the absorption of a photon. Such *photoconversion* between isomers can occur whether the chromophore is free in solution or covalently bound to opsin.

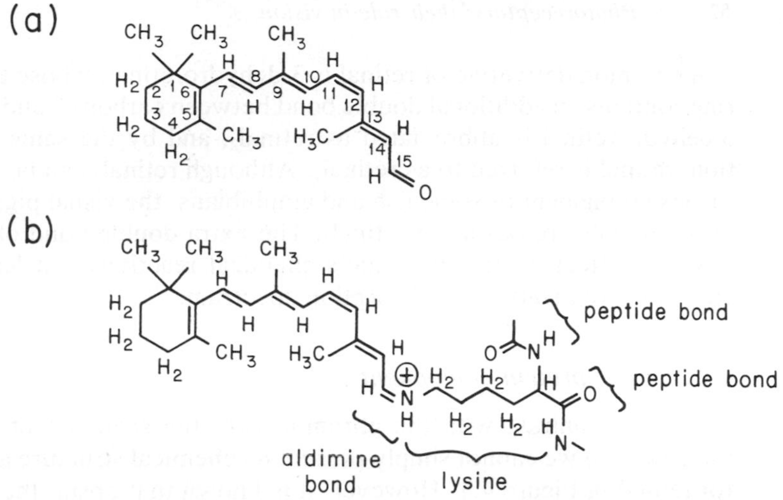

Figure 4.1. (*a*) Retinal, the free chromophore of visual pigments, in its 11-*cis* isomer form. (*b*) The bound chromophore in vertebrate visual pigments. The aldehyde on retinal reacts with the ϵ-amino group of lysine to form an aldimine bond, which subsequently becomes protonated.

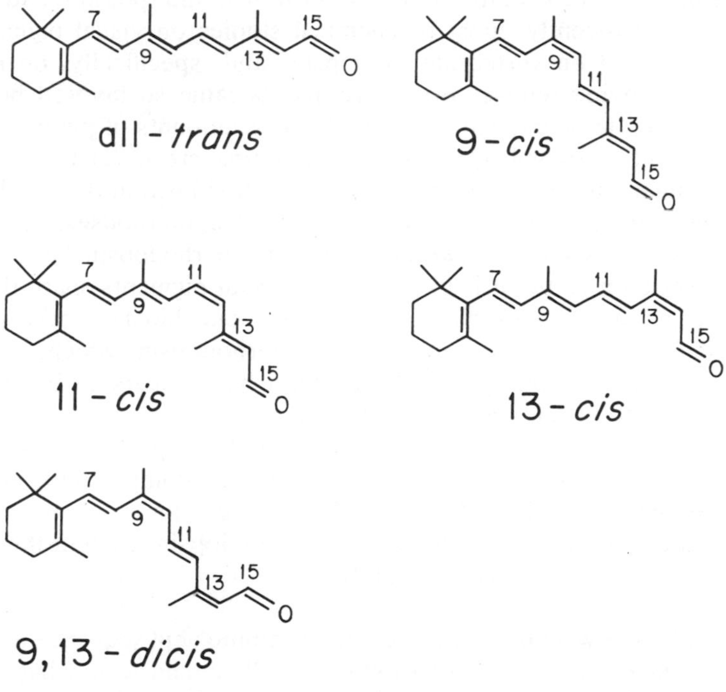

Figure 4.2. Various isomers of retinal. For simplicity, hydrogens are omitted in these structures.

A common derivative of retinal is 3-dehydroretinal, whose β-ionone ring contains an additional double bond between carbons 3 and 4. Often 3-dehydroretinal is abbreviated as $retinal_2$, and by the same convention, retinal is referred to as $retinal_1$. Although $retinal_2$ can be found in the visual pigment of some fish and amphibians, the visual pigments of most animals are based on $retinal_1$. The extra double bond of $retinal_2$ has little effect on the molecule's chemical reactivity but leads to a significant red shift in its absorption spectrum.

4.2.2 The protein component

In contrast with the chromophore, the structure of opsin is unknown, so we cannot simply present its chemical structure as we did for retinal in Figure 4.1. However, it is known that opsin, the apoprotein of all visual pigments, is an intrinsic membrane protein with a single polypeptide chain to which two short oligosaccharide segments are connected. Whereas the chromophore in visual pigments is either $retinal_1$ or $retinal_2$, opsin's structure appears to be less conserved, especially between phylogenetically distant species. Thus visual pigments are isozymes, which are molecules with identical biological functions but with different compositions, and, possibly, structures.

Until recently, most biochemical studies on visual pigments were performed on vertebrate rhodopsins and, specifically, on rhodopsin from bovine retinas. Bovine retinas became so favored because (1) they are large enough to yield adequate amounts of pigment (pigment content is roughly proportional to retina size), (2) they essentially contain only one type of pigment, the rhodopsin in their rods, and (3) they can be routinely obtained from slaughterhouses. Even though most biochemical experiments on animal rhodopsin have been performed on cattle, it is likely that all visual pigments share the general properties of bovine rhodopsin. Lately, some biochemical research has shifted to a related molecule, bacteriorhodopsin, which is a pigment found only within halophilic bacteria but appears to be structurally similar to visual pigments (see Section 4.3).

Complete structural characterization of any protein requires knowledge of its molecular weight, amino acid composition, amino acid sequence, and three-dimensional shape (also known as secondary and tertiary structure). With reference to rhodopsin, each of these properties will be discussed separately.

Molecular weight. Until a complete amino acid sequence is achieved, the molecular weight of rhodopsin will remain somewhat uncertain. This is because all the commonly employed techniques, whether they are based on amino acid analysis, ultracentrifugation, or electrophoresis, are subject to error. The values cited here have been confirmed by several techniques and are likely to be within 20% of the true value. With this note of caution, the molecular weight of bovine rhodopsin can be given as 38,000 (Hubbard, 1954; Daemen et al., 1972; Lewis et al., 1974; Plantner and Kean, 1976); of frog rhodopsin as 40,000 (Robinson et al., 1972); and of squid rhodopsin as 49,000 (Hagins, 1973). Bacteriorhodopsin, with a molecular weight of 25,000, is the smallest pigment. The chromophore, with a molecular weight of about 285, contributes very little to the total weight of the protein complex.

Amino acid composition. The amino acid compositions of several rhodopsins are listed in Table 4.1. Note that the relative ratios of the amino acids and their total number vary markedly among these phylogenetically distant organisms; this variation being the basis for the aforementioned statement that visual pigments are variable in composition. In minor aspects, the data cited in Table 4.1 may be incorrect. Careful experiments, which measured just the cystine content, indicate that each rhodopsin may contain as much as 10 to 12 half-cystines (de Grip et al., 1973; Schwartz et al., 1977).

Amino acid sequence. The complete amino acid sequence of vertebrate rhodopsin still remains to be determined. As of now, only the terminal regions have been sequenced (see Table 4.2). The two carbohydrate chains are attached to the polypeptide near the amino end (Heller, 1968; Fukuda et al., 1979). These side chains are relatively short and are identical in composition: three mannose and three *N*-acetylglucosamine groups. Although most integral membrane proteins are glycosylated, rhodopsin is unusual because its sugar chains are structurally simple and lack sialic acid. The sugar groups, whose specific function is unknown, contribute about 2200 toward the molecular weight of the pigment molecule. As for most intrinsic membrane proteins, rhodopsin's sugar groups are excluded from the cytoplasm; they face either the extracellular space or, in rod disks, the intradiskal space (Röhlich, 1976), which, as recalled, is transiently continuous with extracellular space during disk biogenesis.

Three-dimensional structure. Vertebrate rhodopsin is most likely prolate-shaped, with a major axis of about 75 Å and a minor axis of about 30 Å (Wu and Stryer, 1972). The major axis is perpendicular to the surface of the membrane and parallel to the membrane's lipid chains. Available evidence strongly suggests that it spans the membrane in which it is embedded. With the carboxyl and amino termini on opposite sides of the membrane, the single polypeptide chain must cross the membrane an odd number of times. For favorable hydrophobic interactions between a protein and its adjacent lipid molecules, thermody-

Table 4.1. *Amino acid composition of some visual pigments*

	Bovine rhodopsin			Squid rhodopsin	Bacteriorhodopsin	
Amino acid	Plantner and Kean (1976)	Shichi et al. (1969)[a]	Zorn and Futterman (1971)[a]	Hagins (1973)	Ovchinnikov et al. (1979)	Keefer and Bradshaw (1977)
Polar						
Lys	14	11	12	19	7	6
His	6	5	7	6	0	0
Arg	8	7	7	11	8	7
Asx[b]	24	26	24	32	11	13
Asp	—	—	—	—	8	—
Asn	—	—	—	—	3	—
Thr	26	34	30	16	18	18
Ser	15	21	23	28	14	14
Glx[b]	33	34	32	45	13	14
Glu	—	—	—	—	11	—
Gln	—	—	—	—	2	—
Half-cystine	5	8	8	10	0	0
Nonpolar						
Trp	—	—	—	8	7	7
Pro	22	22	24	41	11	11
Gly	26	28	25	33	25	25
Ala	31	34	29	42	30	29
Val	30	21	26	22	21	20
Met	10	11	12	22	9	8
Ile	20	13	15	36	15	13
Leu	30	27	26	25	34	33
Tyr	16	14	17	20	11	10
Phe	33	29	32	24	13	12
Total	349	—	—	440	247	240

[a] The published data were recalculated for a molecular weight of 38,000.
[b] In most experiments, Asp and Asn could not be separately identified and so are jointly called Asx. Similarly, Glx is a noncommittal form for referring to either Glu or Gln.

namics predicts that a polypeptide must either be an α-helix or a β-structure. Helices are more likely for rhodopsin because both nonresonance Raman spectroscopy (Rothschild et al., 1976) and circular dichroism measurements (Shichi et al., 1969; Shichi and Shelton, 1974; Stubbs et al., 1976) detect extensive helices with little or no β-structures. Apparently, 47 to 60% of all the amino acids of bovine

Table 4.2. *Partial amino acid sequence for bovine rhodopsin.*

Sequence	Structure
Amino terminal with location and composition of carbohydrate side chains[a]	Man (branch) on GlcNAc-GlcNAc-Man-Man-GlcNAc attached to Asn-2; Man (branch) on GlcNAc-GlcNAc-Man-Man-GlcNAc attached to Asn-15 Man | GlcNAc-GlcNAc-Man-Man-GlcNAc Man | | | GlcNAc-GlcNAc-Man-Man-GlcNAc | 10 | 20 (B)Met-Asn-Gly-Thr-Glu-Gly-Pro-Asn-Phe-Tyr-Val-Pro-Phe-Ser-Asn-Lys-Thr-Gly-Val-Val-Arg
Carboxyl terminal[b]	30′ -Arg-Asx-Cys-Met-Val-Thr-Thr-Leu-Cys-Cys-Gly-Lys-Asn-Pro-Leu- 20′ 10′ -Gly-Asp-Asp-Glu-Ala-Ser-Thr-Thr-Val-Ser-Lys-Thr-Glu-Thr-Ser-Gln-Val-Ala-Pro-Ala.

[a] Data from Hargrave and Fong, 1977, and Fukuda et al., 1979. Abbreviations: B, blocked amino terminal; Man, mannose; GlcNAc, *N*-acetylglucosamine. By convention, the numbering of residue locations along the polypeptide chain begins at the amino terminal.
[b] Data from Hargrave and Fong, 1977, and Hargrave et al., 1980. The temporary numbering system for the carboxyl-terminal region uses "primed" numbers and begins at the carboxyl terminal.

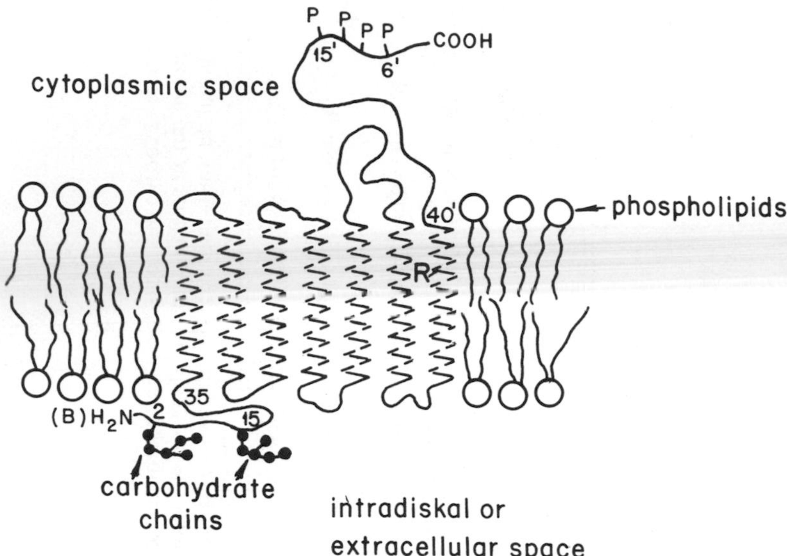

Figure 4.3. Plausible model for the secondary structure of vertebrate rhodopsin. The most probable location of the chromophore is represented by R, and P indicates the location of the amino acid residues that become phosphorylated by a light-induced process. The numbers refer to the location of residues along the sequenced regions of the polypeptide chain. (After Hargrave et al., 1980.)

rhodopsin are within helical regions. Given the number of potential amino acids and an axial distance of 1.5 Å per residue for an α-helix, as many as seven helices could traverse the 40-Å-thick hydrophobic region of a receptor membrane. The lower limit for the number of traverses is three, from proteolytic studies (Fung and Hubbell, 1978*b*). Thus the number of transmembrane helices for vertebrate rhodopsin may be three, five, or seven. Several investigators (Fung and Hubbell, 1978*b;* Hargrave et al., 1980) have presented plausible models for the tertiary structure of bovine rhodopsin. One of these, assuming the seven-helix arrangement, is presented in Figure 4.3. As will be shown in the next section, seven transmembrane helices are known to exist in bateriorhodopsin. It is conceivable that vertebrate rhodopsins and bacteriorhodopsins share similar secondary and tertiary structures.

Retinal–opsin bond. Retinal's covalent bond to opsin is due to a condensation reaction between the aldehyde group on retinal and the ε-amino group on one of opsin's lysine residue (Bownds, 1967; Akhtar et al., 1967). The reaction yields a carbon-nitrogen double-bond linkage (see Figure 4.1), which is called an *aldimine* (for aldehyde and imine), or a *Schiff's base* bond. The reaction is spontaneous, provided that opsin has not been previously denatured. The aldimine bond appears to be universal for all visual pigments studied so far. Sequence analysis on both cattle and pig rhodopsin has revealed that the lysine, which binds retinal, is located about 50 amino acids away from the carboxyl terminal (Wang et al., 1980; Findlay et al., 1981).

4.3 Structure of bacteriorhodopsin

When discussing rhodopsin's structure, mention of bacteriorhodopsin is inevitable even though the latter pigment is found only in halophilic bacteria, in which the presence of visual information processing is debatable. Nevertheless, bacteriorhodopsin must be mentioned because structurally it is very similar to the visual pigments of vertebrates and invertebrates and, more importantly, because its structure is nearly completely characterized. What could not be done for rhodopsin can be done for bacteriorhodopsin: its complete chemical structure can be drawn on paper, just as retinal's structure could be drawn in Figure 4.1.

Bacteriorhodopsin is the first integral membrane protein that has so far been completely sequenced (Ovchinnikov et al., 1979). Its full amino acid sequence is presented in Table 4.3. Henderson and Unwin (1975) determined its three-dimensional structure with an image-reconstruction technique using electron micrographs. The molecule was found to have seven α-helical segments, each of which traverses the membrane nearly at right angles to the membrane surface (Figure 4.4). Using analytical techniques, Engelman et al. (1980) fit the amino acid sequence to the three-dimensional structure and arrived at the most probable way in which the polypeptide backbone is actually folded in the membrane (Figure 4.5). Note that the chromophore, linked to a lysine residue, is near the carboxylic end of the molecule, in analogy with vertebrate rhodopsin. Although the polyene chain of the chromophore makes an angle of about 25° with the plane of the membrane, as determined by linear dichroism measurements (Heyn et al., 1977; Bogomolni et al., 1977), its exact orientation within the plane of the membrane and with respect to the other helices is unknown. The analogy between bacteriorhodopsin and rhodopsin probably ends with their structural similarity and does not extend to their function. On light absorption, bacteriorhodopsin functions as a proton pump (see review by Eisenbach and Caplan, 1979), which is unlikely to be the case for the visual pigments (see Chapter 11).

Table 4.3. *Complete amino acid sequence of bacteriorhodopsin*

(B)[a]Glu - Ala - Gln - Ile - Thr - Gly - Arg - Pro - Glu - Trp - Ile - Trp - Leu - Ala - Leu - Gly - Thr - Ala - Leu - Met-	20
Gly - Leu - Gly - Thr - Leu - Tyr - Phe - Leu - Val - Lys - Gly - Met - Gly - Val - Ser - Asp - Pro - Asp - Ala - Lys-	40
Lys - Phe - Tyr - Ala - Ile - Thr - Thr - Leu - Val - Pro - Ala - Ile - Ala - Phe - Thr - Met - Tyr - Leu - Ser - Met-	60
Leu - Leu - Gly - Tyr - Gly - Leu - Thr - Met - Val - Pro - Phe - Gly - Gly - Glu - Gln - Asn - Pro - Ile - Tyr - Trp-	80
Ala - Arg - Tyr - Ala - Asp - Trp - Leu - Phe - Thr - Thr - Pro - Leu - Leu - Leu - Leu - Asp - Leu - Ala - Leu - Leu-	100
Val - Asp - Ala - Asp - Glu - Gly - Thr - Ile - Leu - Ala - Ile - Val - Gly - Ala - Asp - Gly - Leu - Met - Ile - Gly-	120
Thr - Gly - Leu - Val - Gly - Ala - Leu - Thr - Lys - Val - Tyr - Ser - Tyr - Arg - Phe - Val - Trp - Ala - Ile - Ser-	140
Thr - Ala - Ala - Met - Ser - Tyr - Ile - Leu - Tyr - Val - Leu - Phe - Phe - Gly - Phe - Thr - Ser - Lys - Ala - Glu-	160
Ser - Met - Arg - Pro - Glu - Val - Ala - Ser - Thr - Phe - Lys - Val - Leu - Arg - Asn - Val - Thr - Val - Val - Leu-	180
Trp - Ser - Ala - Tyr - Pro - Val - Val - Trp - Leu - Ile - Gly - Ser - Glu - Gly - Ala - Gly - Ile - Val - Pro - Leu-	200
Asn - Ile - Glu - Thr - Ala - Leu - Phe - Met - Val - Leu - Asp - Val - Ser - Ala - Lys - Val - Gly - Phe - Gly - Leu-	220
Ile - Leu - Leu - Arg - Ser - Arg - Ala - Ile - Phe - Gly - Glu - Ala - Glu - Ala - Pro - Glu - Pro - Ser - Ala - Gly- Asp - Gly - Ala - Ala - Ala - Thr - Ser	240

[a] The amino terminal of the polypeptide chain is blocked by a pyrrole ring and is designated by (B). By convention, the numbering of residue locations along the polypeptide chain begins at the amino terminal.
Source: Ovchinnikov et al., 1979.

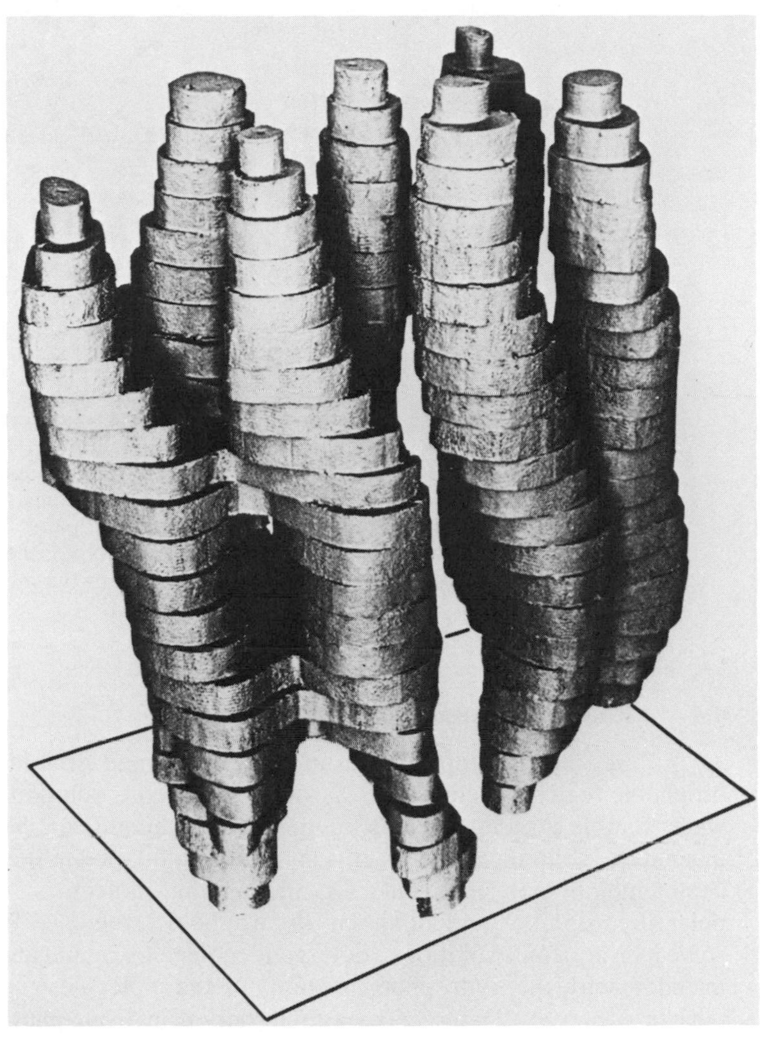

Figure 4.4. A model of the three-dimensional structure of bacteriorhodopsin, based on low-resolution maps of electron-scattering density. The molecule's polypeptide chain is folded into seven α-helices, each of which appears in this model as a vertical stack of round blocks. Each helix traverses the thickness of the membrane so that the ends (on top and bottom of the model) contact the aqueous medium on either side of the membrane and the side of each helix is surrounded by lipid molecules. The molecule has overall dimensions of about 25 × 35 × 45 Å, with the longest dimension perpendicular to the membrane and parallel to the helices. (From Henderson and Unwin, 1975.)

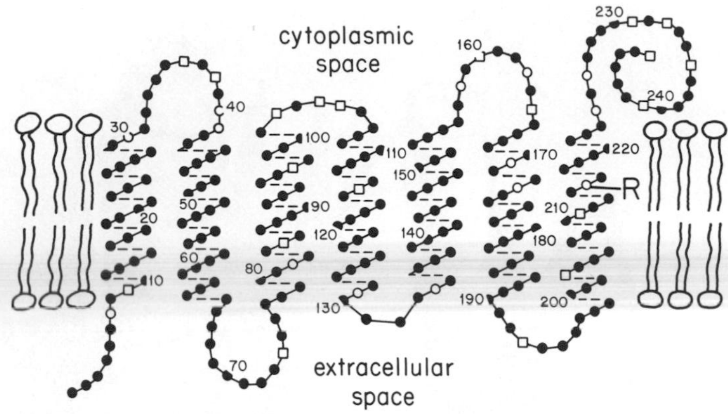

Figure 4.5. Plausible model for the folding of bacteriorhodopsin's polypeptide chain within the membrane. The location of each amino acid is indicated as: ●, if it is uncharged; ○, if positively charged; and □, if negatively charged. Charged residues within the membrane most likely neutralize each other as ion pairs. The location of every tenth amino acid is numbered. Note, the location of the chromophore (R) near the carboxylic end of the molecule. (After Engelman et al., 1980 and Bayley et al., 1981.)

4.4 Rhodopsin extraction from membranes

Because rhodopsin is an integral membrane protein with hydrophobic regions, it cannot be dissolved in aqueous solutions as other water-soluble proteins such as bovine serum albumin can. To study it in solution, solubilizer (detergent) is needed to dissociate the photoreceptor membrane. Detergents are amphipathic molecules, with both polar (hydrophilic) and nonpolar (hydrophobic) regions. When dissolved in aqueous solutions, detergent molecules aggregate to form micelles, with the hydrophobic regions of the molecules forming the micelle's interior. Detergents extract rhodopsin from photoreceptor membranes by incorporating membrane fragments into those micelles. Depending on the detergent and the experimental condition, the solubilized membrane fragments vary in size, with each micelle containing one or possibly several rhodopsins and many lipid molecules. Not all detergents are equally effective in extracting rhodopsin and, more importantly, in extracting it without denaturation. The ideal detergent should not alter rhodopsin's three testable properties:

1. its absorption spectrum,
2. its rate of formation when opsin and 11-*cis* retinal are mixed together, and

3. its thermal stability, as judged by the effect of temperature on its absorption.

Of all the currently used detergents, digitonin is the closest to the ideal because it meets criteria 1 and 2 and only modestly reduces thermal stability. Rhodopsin is so stable within disk membranes that temperatures must exceed 60°C before any thermal effects can be experimentally observed (Hubbard, 1958). If the data obtained at elevated temperatures are extrapolated to body temperature, the rate of thermal bleaching is about 6×10^{-11} $\sec^{-1}$ for cattle rhodopsin, which is equivalent to a decay half-time of 370 yr.

4.5 Absorption spectrum of rhodopsin

The absorption spectrum of rhodopsin is a reflection of retinal's stereochemistry and its covalent linkage to opsin. Although many isomers of retinal can react with opsin, 11-*cis* is the most favored and, as far as is known, is the only isomer found naturally in the primary pigments of photoreceptors, where *primary pigment* refers to the state in which rhodopsin exists in a dark-adapted photoreceptor. As will be discussed in Chapter 6, illumination initiates a series of transient pigment states for which the chromophore assumes the all-*trans* configuration.

The polyene chain contains two single bonds, at carbons 6 and 12, about which rotations are sterically possible. Because the energy barrier separating the conformations obtained by such rotations is less than the thermal energies available at normal temperatures, 11-*cis* retinal in solution exists as an equilibrium mixture of several conformers (Figure 4.6). However, when reacted with bovine opsin, retinal assumes a single conformation: 6s-*cis,* 11-*cis* with all the remaining bonds in *trans* conformation. It is not yet known how universal this conformation is for vertebrate and invertebrate visual pigments.

Although exceptions exist, color is one of the characteristic properties of visual pigments. By themselves, opsin and the chromophore appear colorless to the human eye. (To be exact, concentrated solutions of retinal are pale yellow because retinal absorbs somewhat at the extreme blue end of the visible spectrum.) However, when bound to each other, the combination typically absorbs visible light.

The effect of bovine opsin on the absorption spectrum of retinal is illustrated in Figure 4.7. As shown, opsin does not absorb at all beyond 280 nm, that is, beyond the absorption band for the common aromatic amino acids of tryptophan, tyrosine, and phenylalanine. Free retinal's preferential absorption at 380 nm is closer to, but still outside, the visible range. With cattle rhodopsin, however, the absorption band

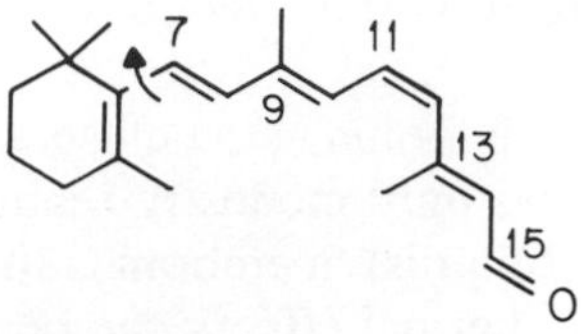

Figure 4.6. Some of the various conformations of 11-*cis* retinal arising from rotations about single bonds. For simplicity, hydrogens are omitted in these structures.

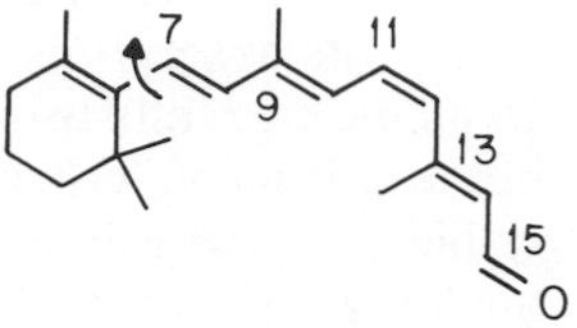

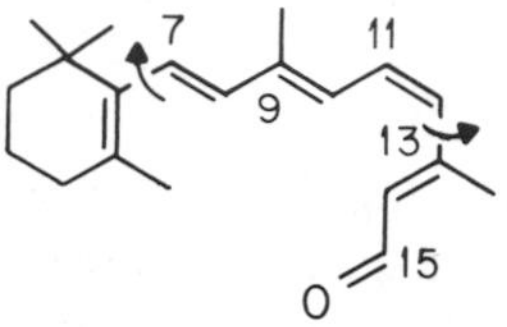

moves into the visible, with the spectral position of its peak sensitivity (or λ_{max}) at 500 nm. The spectral location of λ_{max} varies greatly among species, ranging from the blue to the red end of the spectrum. With its absorption peak near 500 nm, a wavelength that is bluish green, bovine rhodopsin is typical of most vertebrate pigments found in mammalian and amphibian rods.

Understanding the molecular mechanism whereby vertebrate opsin shifts the chromophore's λ_{max} into the visible has been one of the primary goals of visual chemistry. In spectral terms, a shift toward longer wavelengths where photons are less energetic simply means that the electrons in the polyene chain are delocalized, occupying shallower potential wells so that less energy is required to excite them. It is now agreed that the Schiff's base linkage together with its protonation can yield a red shift of as much as 50 to 100 nm (Kropf and Hubbard, 1958). Kropf and Hubbard suggested that further red shifts could arise if electrostatic interactions occurred between the chromophore and the opsin. Recently, Honig and co-workers (1979) demonstrated the existence of such charge interactions using spectroscopic and theoretical analysis of visual pigment analogs. They suggested that two negative charges from the protein are in close proximity to retinal's polyene chain (Figure 4.8). Spatial variation between the charges and the chro-

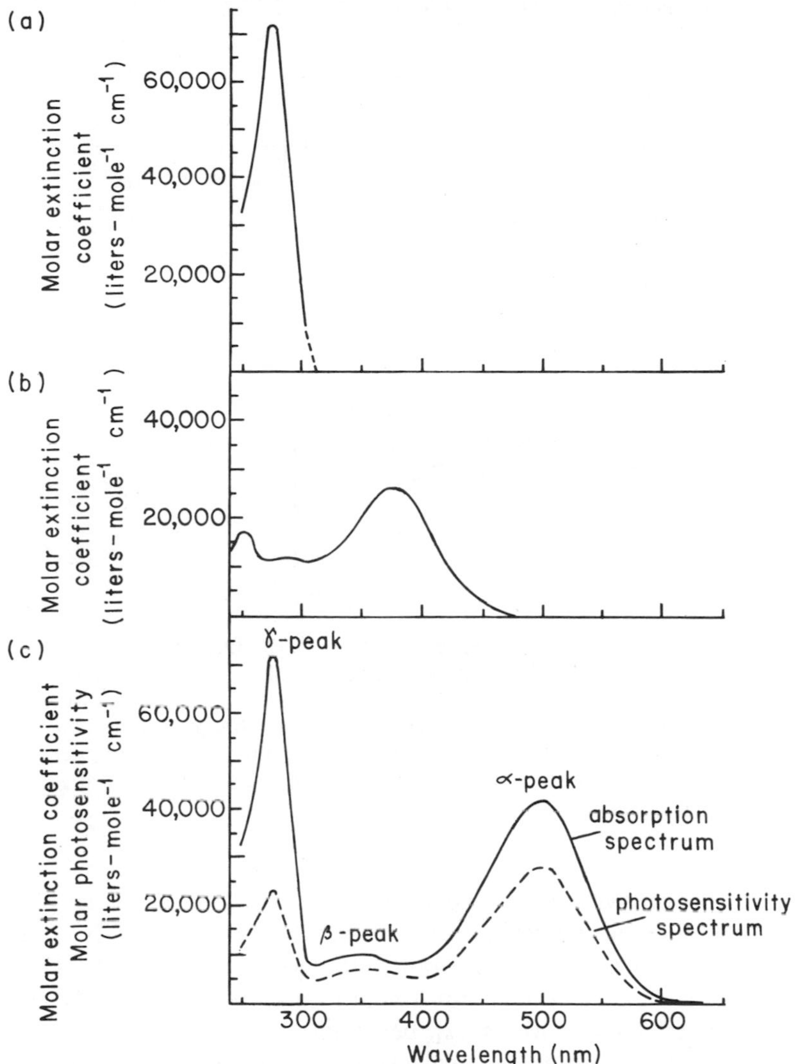

Figure 4.7. Absorption spectra of rod opsin, free retinal, and their reaction product, rhodopsin. On the ordinate is plotted the molar extinction coefficient. (After Ebrey and Honig, 1975.) (*a*) The opsin spectrum was based on the γ-peak of rhodopsin. Its absorption beyond 300 nm was made to fit the absorption profile of the absorbing cyclic amino acids. Such a reconstruction is necessary because purified opsin preparations usually contain irremovable chromophore contaminants that strongly absorb in this part of the spectrum. (*b*) 11-*cis* retinal dissolved in ethanol. (*c*) Cattle rhodopsin solubilized with the detergent ammonyx-LO. Both its absorption spectrum (solid line) and photosensitivity spectrum (dashed line), as derived from the data of Goodeve et al. (1942), Kropf (1967), and Dartnall (1968), are shown for the sake of comparison.

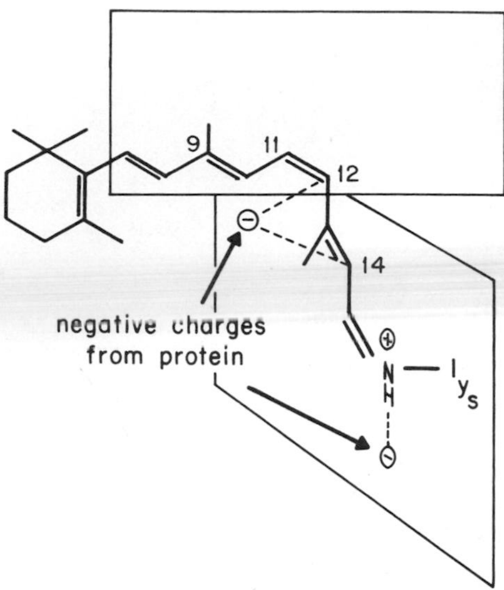

Figure 4.8. A plausible model for electrostatic interaction between the chromophore and the protein component of rhodopsin. The relative positions of the two planes within which the atoms of the polyene chain lie are shown. Two negatively charged amino acid side chains interact with the chromophore, one at the protonated Schiff's base and one at carbons 12 and 14. (After Honig et al., 1979.)

mophore apparently explains the wavelength variation of visual pigments, including the spectral intermediates following photoactivation.

Not all visual pigments show a red-shifted spectral sensitivity. One of the three rhodopsins commonly found in insects preferentially absorbs at about 350 nm, with its λ_{max} being about 30 nm further into the UV than that of free retinal. As was shown in *Ascalaphus macaronius* (Schwemer et al., 1971) and *Deilephila elpenor* (Schwemer and Paulsen, 1973), these UV-sensitive rhodopsins also consist of 11-*cis* retinal, which is covalently bound to opsin. As a result, the chromophore–opsin interactions in these pigments may be significantly different than in the more commonly studied rhodopsins.

The three characteristic peaks of rhodopsin's absorption spectrum are usually designated by the initial letters of the Greek alphabet (see Figure 4.7). Of these, only the γ-peak is due to protein absorption. The electronic transition moments, representing absorptions in the α- and β-peaks, have been the subject of several investigations. The α-peak results from a transition moment that induces electronic oscillations along the entire length of the conjugated bonds. Because the polyene chain for 11-*cis* retinal is bent, the orientation of this transition moment is at some intermediate angle to the two linear segments, its exact direction being unknown. Thus, the orientation of the chromophore cannot be accurately deduced even if the angle of its transition moment vector with respect to a specific direction is known. The situation is simpler for bacteriorhodopsin, where the transition moment vector coincides with the straight polyene chain of the all-*trans* isomer. Interestingly, linear dichroism measurements indicate that the angle between the plane of the membrane and the transition moment vector is very similar in both vertebrates and halophilic bacteria. The β-peak represents transition moments that involve only partial oscillations along the bent polyene chain; the direction of their moments remains very uncertain.

4.6 Physical significance of absorption spectra

The fraction of light absorbed by an infinitely thin layer of pigmented solution is proportional to the pigment concentration and to the distance covered by the light rays as they pass through the solution. This physical property, true for all pigmented solutions, is mathematically expressed as

$$-dI/I = \alpha c\, dx \tag{4.1}$$

where I is the incident light intensity, dI the transmitted intensity minus the incident intensity, α the proportionality factor, which is wavelength-dependent and has units of square centimeters, c the pigment concentration in molecules per cubic centimeter, and dx the path length in centimeters. The left side of Equation (4.1) is equal to the fraction of photons absorbed and the right side to the product of α and the number of molecules within the beam's cross-sectional area ($c\, dx$). The right-hand side of the equation can also be thought of as the number of molecules multiplied by the probability that a single molecule will absorb a photon. Thus, α is actually the *absorption cross section* of a single molecule, and it is an intrinsic molecular property. Because solutions are not infinitely thin, Equation (4.1) needs to be integrated to be of practical use. With additional dimensional and logarithmic conversions, the solution for the fraction of transmitted light becomes

$$I_t/I_i = 10^{-\epsilon cl} \tag{4.2}$$

where I_t is the transmitted light intensity, I_i the incident light intensity, ϵ the *molar extinction coefficient* in liters per mole-centimeter, c the concentration in moles per liter, and l the solution thickness, or path length, in centimeters. Equation (4.2) is commonly known as the *Beer–Lambert law*. As before, only ϵ is wavelength-dependent among the three independent variables. For the sake of convenience, photochemists transform Equation (4.2) by defining *absorbance* A as $\log(I_i/I_t)$. (Absorbance is really a misnomer because it is not directly related to the fraction of light absorbed but rather to that transmitted.) Its substitution into Equation (4.2) yields

$$A = \epsilon c l \tag{4.3}$$

Absorbance, also called *optical density,* is a dimensionless number and is regularly measured with a common laboratory spectrophotometer. Its variation with wavelength is known as the *absorbance spectrum.*

Performing the mathematical manipulations shows that the molar extinction coefficient times a constant, 3.8×10^{-21} cm^3-mole liter^{-1}, is numerically equal to the molecule's absorption cross section. Thus, the molar extinction coefficient, an intrinsic molecular property, also reflects the probability of photon absorption. In essence, the absorbance spectrum then gives the *relative* probability of photon absorption as a function of wavelength. As Figure 4.7 illustrates, the extinction coefficient of rhodopsin at its λ_{max} is about 42,000 liters cm^{-1}-mole^{-1} (Shichi et al., 1969; Daemen et al., 1970; Bridges, 1971). This value appears to be universally applicable for all retinal$_1$-based visual pigments, irrespective of their origin or λ_{max}, and from it the absorption cross section of a single rhodopsin molecule in solution can be calculated to be 1.6 Å^2 (Dartnall, 1972).

Visual scientists measuring receptor function are less interested in the intrinsic properties of rhodopsin than in the overall properties of a cell. For their purposes, the fraction of incident light that is absorbed (I_a/I_i) is more important than absorbance because it is the light that is absorbed which is chemically effective. Starting from Equation (4.2), I_a/I_i can be derived and given as

$$I_a/I_i = 1 - (I_t/I_i) = 1 - 10^{-\epsilon c l} = 1 - 10^{-A} \tag{4.4}$$

This ratio is known as *absorptance* (often confused with and even sometimes called absorbance) and its variation with wavelength as the *absorptance spectrum.* It is this spectrum, rather than the absorbance spectrum, that is related to the action spectrum commonly measured by physiologists. Note that absorptance is a logarithmic, not a linear, function of the three independent variables. Only when the pigment concentration is infinitely dilute and the path length infinitely short does absorptance exactly equal absorbance. Because infinitely dilute and infinitely short conditions are rarely encountered, the shape of an absorptance spectrum can deviate from that of an absorbance spectrum. As concentration and path length increases in the product ϵcl, the absorptance spectrum becomes increasingly broader. This is the reason why any pigment can look black if it is concentrated enough. On the other hand, the shape of the absorbance curve is invariant with concentration and thickness. This is why it is so useful in the identification of chemical compounds. Microspectrophotometric data from vertebrate receptors indicate relatively high absorbances along the outer segment's axis. For human rods and toad red rods, respective absorbances are 0.48 and 1.0, with corresponding absorptances being 0.67 and 0.90 (Bowmaker and Dartnall, 1980; Harosi, 1975). (Note that these visual cells absorb 67 and 90% of any axially incident light.) Given the recorded absorbances, the action spectra of these cells should be significantly broadened (refer to Figure 5.4).

4.7 Quantum efficiency of photoactivation or bleaching

Many pigments in nature are stable to illumination. When pigments in artist paints or in flower petals absorb a photon, the absorbed energy is quickly transformed into vibrational energy (heat), leaving the pigment unaffected in its structure and spectral property. Visual pigments, however, are photolabile – light absorption transforms them into different spectral states. The initial step of this transformation is usually called *photoactivation,* or photoexcitation. Photoactivation initiates a sequence of dark reactions, which do not require light and which ultimately terminate with products that are stable with time. These end products may be colorless (i.e., bleached), as for vertebrates, or may remain colored, as is the case for invertebrates. The probability that the absorption of a photon initiates photoactivation is expressed as the *quantum efficiency of photoactivation* and for vertebrates, where the photoactivated molecules eventually bleach, is also known as *quantum efficiency of bleaching*. This probability is defined as

$$\begin{matrix}\text{quantum}\\\text{efficiency}\\\text{for photo}\\\text{activation}\end{matrix} = \frac{\text{number of photoactivated molecules}}{\text{number of molecules that absorbed a photon}} \tag{4.5}$$

At any wavelength, this ratio is numerically equal to the molar photosensitivity divided by the molar extinction coefficient. Photosensitivity measurements employ the same techniques as absorption measurements and operationally involve recording the temporal absorbance decrease when a rhodopsin solution is illuminated with monochromatic light. Because quantum efficiency is unitless, both *molar photosensitivity* (essentially the probability that rhodopsin is photoactivated by an incident photon) and *molar extinction coefficient* (essentially the probability that rhodopsin has absorbed an incident photon) share the same units of liters per mole-centimeter. Their numerical values are plotted together as a function of wavelength in Figure 4.7. Quantum efficiency throughout the α- and β-bands was found to be wavelength-independent and to be equal to about 0.7 (Goodeve et al., 1942; Dartnall, 1968). Thus the probability of photoactivation with visible light is about 70%. The remaining 30% of the absorbed photons produce only heat; they do not lead to the formation of bathorhodopsin, which is the product of photoactivation (see Chapter 6). The quantum efficiency of photoactivation is practically the same for all visual pigments, whether based on $retinal_1$ or $retinal_2$. Although quantum efficiency drops in the UV, it remains relatively high. Apparently UV energy absorbed by the protein is somehow transferred to the chromophore by an intramolecular process (Kropf, 1967).

A constant quantum efficiency throughout the visible range has great implications for receptor physiology. The immediate conclusion is that *once absorbed, every photon in the visible range is equally likely to photoactivate rhodopsin.* Because it is the photoactivated state of rhodopsin that initiates the dark reactions of phototransduction and leads to the photoresponse, the quantum efficiency for photoreceptor excitation should also be constant throughout the visible spectrum. This statement is commonly referred to as the *univariance principle* (Naka and Rushton, 1966). To quote Naka and Rushton (p. 538): "The signals from each [visual pigment or receptor] depend only upon the rate at which it is effectively catching quanta; it does not depend upon the associated wavelength." Though the coupling between photoactivated rhodopsin and photoresponse generation need not be perfect, experimental data indicate a nearly 100% linkage (see Chapter 9).

This is an appropriate point at which to expound further on the subject of light detectors. All detectors absorb photons and at any wavelength produce signals in proportion to the rate of absorbed photons. However, when their response to different wavelengths is considered, they can be grouped into two classes: if their signal amplitude is proportional to the number of absorbed photons, independent of the photon's energy, then they are *quantum detectors;* if, however, their signal amplitude is proportional to the photon's energy, then they are *thermal detectors* (for definitions see, e.g., Jacobs, 1978). Signal amplitude is independent of wavelength for the former and inversely proportional to wavelength for the latter, when the rate of absorbed photons is constant throughout the spectrum. These considerations require that when the spectral response of quantum detectors is measured, the correct units for stimulus intensity be in photon flux density rather than in energy flux density. On the basis of the previous discussion on quantum efficiency of bleaching, photoreceptors clearly belong to the class of quantum detectors.

4.8 Dartnall's relationship and his nomogram

Absorption spectra can be plotted either as a function of wavelength (in nanometers) or as a function of wave number (in reciprocal centimeters) or frequency (in hertz). Dartnall (1953) discovered that when the α-bands of several detergent-solubilized rhodopsins are plotted on a wave number scale, their shape is nearly constant, irrespective of the location of their λ_{max}. This constancy of shape made it possible for Dartnall to construct a nomogram with which the entire absorption band of any visual pigment could be predicted once its λ_{max} was known. Dartnall based his analysis on rather limited data obtained from a handful of species. Subsequently, Bridges (1967) and Munz and Schwanzara (1967) demonstrated that the absorption bands of retinal$_2$-based pigments, which Dartnall did not consider, are broader than that predicted by the Dartnall nomogram. With even more numerous and more accurate data, it was recently realized that, contrary to Dartnall's initial conclusion, the shape of the α-band systematically varies with λ_{max} (Ebrey and Honig, 1977). The variations are so small, however, that the classical nomograms are still valid for pigments with λ_{max} between 500 and 550 nm.

Nomograms have been and shall remain invaluable tools in the analysis of visual pigment spectra. For example, rarely can electrophysiologists obtain enough data points with sufficient accuracy to generate the entire action spectrum of their impaled receptor. With their few points and the nomograms, they can accurately deduce the λ_{max} of their visual pigment and determine whether it contains retinal$_1$ or retinal$_2$. (As will be discussed in the next chapter, caution must be exercised, however, when the nomogram is employed in such a manner.)

4.9 Visual pigment nomenclature

It may seem strange that the fundamental topic of visual pigment nomenclature should be discussed so late in the book. Its discussion has been deferred until now partly because some knowledge about pigment structure is necessary and partly because the naming of visual pigments is mired with confusions and inconsistencies. Rather than present their historical origin and background (see the review by Wald, 1953), the various terminologies currently in use will simply be enumerated.

1. Currently rhodopsin has two meanings, one general and one specific. In its general sense, rhodopsin refers to any primary visual pigment that consists of $retinal_1$ or $retinal_2$ bound to opsin. Because rhodopsins are isozymes that may vary considerably in their structure, they should always be named for the animal of origin, such as cattle rhodopsin, bacteriorhodopsin, or squid rhodopsin. In its specific sense, rhodopsin refers to a subset of vertebrate pigments, which will be described next.

2. Based on Wald's proposal (e.g., Wald, 1953; Wald et al., 1953), the nomenclature for the primary visual pigments of vertebrates is the following:

rod opsin + $retinal_1$ → rhodopsin
rod opsin + $retinal_2$ → porphyropsin
cone opsin + $retinal_1$ → iodopsin
cone opsin + $retinal_2$ → cyanopsin

Note that this nomenclature is based solely on composition and not on subjective color sense or λ_{max}. According to this scheme, all human cone pigments are iodopsins because they contain only $retinal_1$. Similarly, the pigments in goldfish cones are cyanopsins because they are solely based on $retinal_2$.

3. Vertebrate cone pigments are further characterized on the basis of their peak spectral sensitivity λ_{max}. Depending on the location of their λ_{max}, the three commonly encountered cone pigments are referred to as blue-, green-, or red-sensitive cones. Such color designations are actually accurate only for those few animals whose λ_{max} values are indeed located within the appropriately designated region of the spectrum. For instance, this is true of goldfish, whose respective peak sensitivities are at 453, 533, and 620 nm. However, such color names misrepresent the λ_{max} values for most other species, including those of humans.

4. Vertebrate rod pigments are also subdivided on the basis of their spectral location. However, out of historical inertia and to the confusion of the uninitiated, the color attributed to them is based on transmission rather than on preferential absorption as with cones. Thus, frog rods that contain a rhodopsin with a λ_{max} of 502 nm in the blue-green region are called "red" rods, and those with a blue-sensitive pigment (λ_{max} = 433 nm) are named "green" rods.

5. All this confusion on nomenclature is eliminated with Dartnall's (1952) simple, albeit less colorful, notation. According to the com-

monly employed version of his scheme, primary visual pigments are identified by the letter P or R (for photopigment or rhodopsin, respectively), by their λ_{max} in nanometers, and by the subscript 1 or 2, which refers, respectively, to the retinal$_1$ or retinal$_2$ nature of the chromophore. According to this notation, rhodopsin from frog red rods is R502$_1$.

In using the preceding nomenclatures, the same eclectic usage that is currently practiced in the literature will be followed in this book. Visual pigments, in general, will be called rhodopsins. Whenever Wald's specific meaning is meant, the visual pigment will be referred to as vertebrate rhodopsin or will be identified with the vertebrate's name.

4.10 Summary

Rhodopsins are intrinsic membrane proteins composed of a small chromophore and a large glycoprotein, covalently linked to each other with a one-to-one stoichiometry. The spectral property of the pigment is predominantly determined by the chromophore's structure and by the chromophore's interaction with the protein. Although large variations may occur in the molecular structure of rhodopsins from phylogenetically distant species, it is currently thought that at least in visual photoreceptors they share the same biological activity.

5 Color vision and polarization detection

How does the visual system make use of the absorption properties of rhodopsin to detect the spectral composition, degree of polarization, and intensity of light? The remainder of this book attempts to give the answer to this question. The parameters to be considered in this chapter are light's spectral composition and degree of polarization, the perception of which are called color vision and polarization detection, respectively. Though the detection of light's intensity also depends on the pigment's absorption characteristics, its discussion is postponed to subsequent chapters because it requires additional knowledge about the specific effects of photon absorption, none of which are necessary to understand the underlying mechanism that makes the detection of the other two parameters possible.

Almost all our knowledge about color vision and polarization detection is based on experiments that employ either photometric or nonphotometric techniques to measure the in situ properties of visual pigments. Photometric measurements usually rely on a special instrument called a microspectrophotometer, which is similar to the common laboratory spectrophotometer except that its measuring beam passes through a light microscope where it is focused down to an area of a few square microns. Entire photoreceptors or distinct subcellular regions, such as outer segments, can be positioned into the beam for analysis. Nonphotometric measurements utilize the techniques of electrophysiology and, in the case of human perception, psychophysics. The discrepancies that sometimes develop between the two methods of analysis arise from the fact that photometric measurements yield information only about the visual pigment, whereas the nonphotometric measurements depend in addition on receptor physiology and, in the case of psychophysics, also on processing by central neurons.

5.1 Color vision

That artists could generate all the colors of the visible spectrum by mixing in various proportions only three colors of paint (blue,

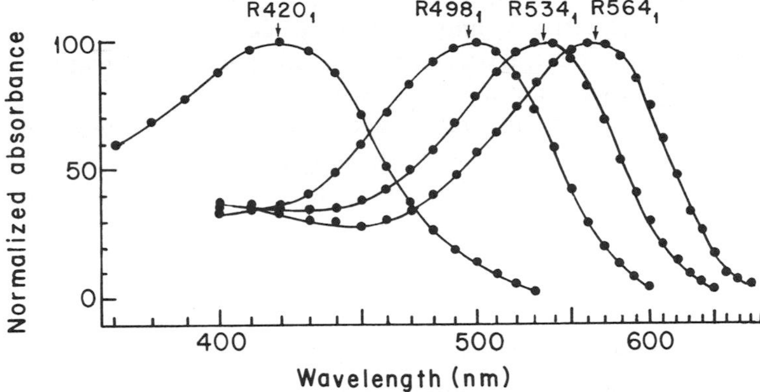

Figure 5.1. Relative absorption spectra of human visual pigments, plotted on a frequency scale that shows only the corresponding wavelengths. The maximal absorbance of the pigments is set to 100 and each pigment is identified by its λ_{max}, the wavelength at which maximal absorption occurs. $R498_1$ is human rhodopsin and is found only in rods. The remaining pigments belong to the three classes of cones, which are called blue-absorbing ($R420_1$), green-absorbing ($R534_1$), and red-adsorbing ($R564_1$). Of all the pigments, the λ_{max} placement of $R420_1$ remains the most uncertain. (After Bowmaker and Dartnall, 1980.)

yellow, and red) has intrigued observers for centuries. Though many attempted to provide a rational explanation for this perceptual phenomenon (a good historical account is given by Brindley, 1970), Young was the first to consider seriously the physical nature of light and to propose in 1802 a theory that has stood the test of time. Young suggested that the human retina contains three different kinds of "sensitive particles," each maximally, but not exclusively, sensitive to different regions of the visible spectrum. Young's *trichromatic theory of human color vision* lacked ultimate proof until it was finally validated by two independent research groups (Marks et al., 1964; Brown and Wald, 1964). Young's particles are, of course, the visual pigments of which, in humans, there are three different kinds segregated into separate cones. The spectral sensitivity of the three classes of human cone receptors is illustrated in Figure 5.1. Though color vision in humans is primarily, if not solely, mediated by cones, the spectral sensitivity of the human rod is also given in Figure 5.1 for the sake of comparison. Note that in contrast with cones, all human rods contain the same pigment.

The data on cones in Figure 5.1 were obtained by microspectrophotometry and could not have been easily obtained with nonphotometric techniques. This is because primate receptors are extremely difficult to impale with microelectrodes, and psychophysical measurements are hindered by extensive central processing. In fact, psychophysical techniques isolate, not three, but as many as seven distinct spectral sensitivity functions (see the review by Rodieck, 1973). Standard biochemical techniques of extraction with detergents are equally useless because cone pigments cannot be readily separated from each other and because detergents readily denature them.

5.1.1 Conditions for color vision

The most fundamental requirement for color vision is the presence of at least two spectrally distinct classes of photoreceptors. Being quantum detectors, photoreceptors generate signals in proportion to the number of absorbed photons. Changes in absorption rate can occur either because intensity is varied or because absorption probability is altered owing to a shift in wavelength. An individual receptor cannot simultaneously transmit information about intensity and wavelength. *To detect color, at least two photoreceptors belonging to different spectral classes need to be excited.* It is not enough that the receptors contain different pigments; they must also operate within the same range of ambient illumination. For example, humans lacking two of their cone classes would be completely color-blind under photopic conditions even though, in addition to their single-cone class, they would still possess a spectrally distinct class of rods. This is the reason why the mere presence of cones in a retina cannot ever be taken as a sufficient criteria for color vision. Of course, a further requirement for color vision is a central processing mechanism that distinguishes among the differentially excited receptor classes. Nonprimate mammals, such as rats, cattle, dogs, and cats, are essentially color-blind even though their rod-dominated retinas contain some cones.

As is well known, humans lack the ability to perceive colors under scotopic conditions because only rods are active under those conditions and because all human rods contain the same visual pigment. Thus, the spectral sensitivity of scotopic vision presented in Figure 1.2*b* is a reflection of rod rhodopsin. It is expected that in the mesopic range of intensities (see Table 1.2) color vision by extrafoveal regions, where both rods and cones are present, should be mediated by all four retinal pigments. However, retinal processing in humans is such that the predicted tetrachromaticity is very difficult to demonstrate (Brindley, 1970, p. 205). As in the photopic range, color vision at mesopic intensities appears to be cone-dominated. Our state of light adaptation does not modify our sense of color; quantitatively the same color matches are produced, irrespective of ambient light intensities.

Because, morphologically, the three classes of human cones are indistinguishable, neither the relative number of the three cone types nor their exact distribution across the retina are known. Psychophysical studies, however, indicate that the blue-sensitive cones are partially or completely absent within a 30′ region at the very center of the fovea. Thus, depending on the region of illumination, the spectral sensitivity of the eye varies. The spectral sensitivity of photopic vision, illustrated in Figure 1.2*b*, was based on measurements taken at the fovea with relatively large retinal fields. It therefore represents some type of combined activity by the three cone receptors.

5.1.2 Some aspects of human color vision

The physiology of human color vision, its capabilities and limitations, ultimately rests on the three types of cones that humans possess. The relative excitation of these cones explains most of the salient features of both normal and abnormal color vision. Whenever incident light excites all three cones more or less equally, we see the color white. If preferential absorption occurred, say, within the red-sensitive receptors, we would identify the incident light as red. Its hue would depend on the light's spectral purity, that is, on the relative excitation of the remaining types of cones. The science of color vision is a vast discipline that is beyond the scope of this book (for recent reviews, see Brindley, 1970; Rodieck, 1973; Hurvich, 1981). Two of its topics, nevertheless, will be briefly mentioned here because they provide the major basis for the success of the trichromatic theory.

a. *Color matching*. The underlying principle behind color matching is that the sensation of any color (whether it is evoked by monochromatic light or by a spectral mixture) depends primarily on the relative excitation of the three spectrally different cones. Thus, with minor exceptions, the color of any wavelength of light can be exactly matched by the suitable combination of three monochromatic beams, whose wavelengths and intensities are independently varied. Note that this means that the eye can confuse stimuli whose wavelength compositions are drastically different. It just does not function as a wavelength analyzer. (In contrast, the ear does. A pure tone could never be "matched" by or confused with a chord of other frequencies, irrespective of how many notes it contained.) In spite of its apparent limitations, the human eye can detect (though not quantitate) very subtle differences in the spectral reflectance of illuminated objects. In the central region of the visible spectrum, humans can discriminate among monochromatic beams whose wavelengths differ as little as 1 nm. This is why, for humans, a rigorous count of perceptually distinct hues easily exceeds thousands. It is tempting to derive quantitatively the results of the color-matching experiments from basic principles, that is, from the relative spectral sensitivity of the three cones in Figure 5.1. However, these experimental data are insufficient by themselves. Additional factors, such as pigment density within each receptor, receptor density within the retina, and, most importantly, type of central processing, must be considered for any successful quantitative description. That color perceptions do not always correspond to the actual spectral distribution of incident photons (Land, 1977) illustrates the overriding importance of central processing.

b. *Abnormal color vision.* Optical measurements and psychophysical measurements have clearly established that most color blindness in humans occurs because one or more of the cone classes is missing, is underrepresented, or has modified spectral sensitivity. In its most frequent form, the form that is sex-linked and observed primarily in males, color-blind individuals easily confuse the colors in the long-wavelength region of the spectrum. Optical measurements on foveal cones (Rushton, 1963; 1965) showed that such people possess only two types of cones; in effect, they lack either the red-sensitive or the green-sensitive cones.

5.1.3 Spectral types in selected organisms

Many organisms besides the primates are capable of color vision. The receptor spectral types in some of these organisms are illustrated in Figure 5.2. The data on frogs are noteworthy because they demonstrate that cones and rods need not possess different types of visual pigments. Note also that in frogs there are two classes of rods; the so-called green rods with $R432_1$, and the red rods with $R502_1$. Insect eyes are characteristically dominated by three types of rhodopsins, maximally sensitive to the green (about 525 nm), to the blue (about 440 nm), and to the UV (about 350 nm). Butterflies, the only exception known so far, possess a fourth pigment whose λ_{max} is near 610 nm (Bernard, 1979). Though all rhodopsins are sensitive to UV-light (humans without their lenses can see and even read in UV), rhodopsins with peak sensitivity in the UV have thus far been demonstrated only in insects and, as far as it is known, are absent in mammals. They may be present in birds because exceptional UV sensitivity can be behaviorally demonstrated in pigeons (Kreithen and Eisner, 1978) and hummingbirds (Goldsmith, 1980).

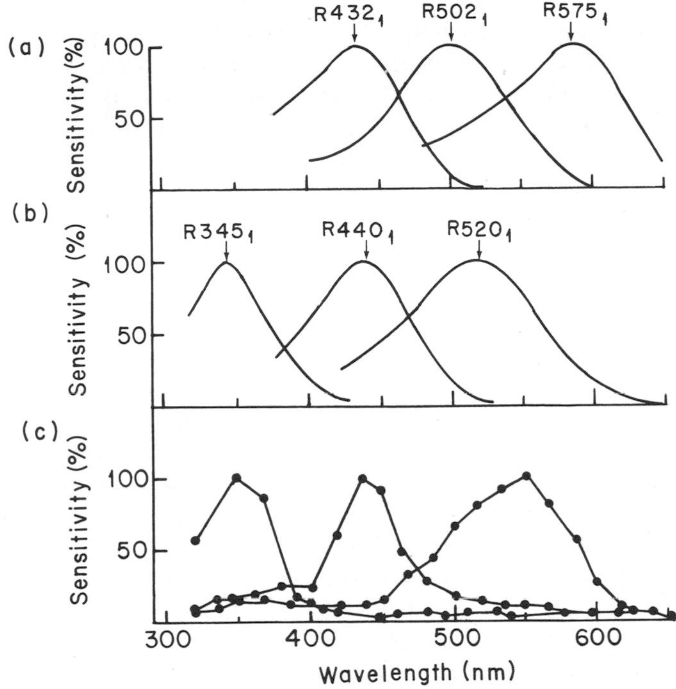

Figure 5.2. Normalized spectral sensitivities of the different classes of receptors found within the eyes of three organisms. (*a*) Normalized absorption spectra for the visual pigments of frog (*Rana pipiens*), as measured by microspectrophotometry. Each visual pigment is identified by its λ_{max}. Rods contain either $R432_1$ or $R502_1$, and the pigment in cones is either $R502_1$ or $R575_1$. (After Liebman and Entine, 1968.) (*b*) Normalized absorption spectra for the visual pigments of the moth (*Deilaphila elpenor*), as based on digitonin extracts from 100 moths. Each visual pigment is identified by its λ_{max}. (After Schwemer and Paulsen, 1973.) (*c*) Normalized action spectra of the receptors of the worker honeybee (*Apis mellifera*), as obtained by intracellular recordings. The individual spectra represent the average behavior of the receptors that showed minimal inter-receptor coupling. Such coupling is especially evident between the UV- and green-sensitive cells. (After Menzel and Blakers, 1976.)

It is interesting to note that polarization detection by bees and other insects (to be discussed subsequently) is primarily, if not solely, mediated by UV receptors (von Frisch, 1967; von Helverson and Edrich, 1974). One would expect that cells employed to detect skylight's polarization would be optimally sensitive either to skylight's predominant wavelength or failing that, to the wavelength where polarization is the greatest. However, such a predicted match does not occur. In terms of incident photons, skylight's intensity peaks at about 450 nm, far from the λ_{max} of UV receptors. Furthermore, skylight's polarization in the UV is usually less than in the visible (cf. Sekera as quoted by von Frisch, 1967, p. 382, and the review by Waterman, 1981).

5.1.4 *Number of pigments per receptor*

On the basis of extensive microspectrophotometric data performed on many species, it appears that as a general rule any given receptor contains only one type of visual pigment. Mixtures rarely occur. Exceptions to this generalization are those organisms (amphibians and fish) that switch from a vitamin A_1-based to an A_2-based pigment during metamorphosis or development. The visual pigments based on these two chromophores may coexist within the same outer segment throughout the transition period and in fish may even persist into adulthood (Bridges, 1972; Loew and Dartnall, 1976; Levine and MacNichol, 1979). Receptors have little control over the type of chromophore that their opsins pick up. It is primarily, if not solely, determined by the pigment epithelium, which supplies the chromophores to the receptors and which contains the necessary biochemical machinery to regenerate the chromophores in large quantities (see Chapter 6). The visual cells, however, do control the type of opsin they synthesize, and on the basis of current data, each receptor appears to manufacture only one type of opsin.

Though only one type of rhodopsin may exist in a receptor, nonrhodopsin pigments can be present. Their presence can significantly modify the cell's spectral sensitivity, as the two following examples illustrate:

(a) The photoreceptors of flies, spiders, etc., exhibit action spectra with two spectral maxima of similar amplitude, one around 500 nm and one in the UV at 360 nm (DeVoe, 1972; Horridge and Mimura, 1975). Comparably sized dual peaks are inconsistent with the absorption spectrum of rhodopsin, whose photosensitivity at 360 nm is only about 20% of its maximum value at 500 nm (see Figure 4.7). Based on microspectrophotometric observations, Kirschfeld et al. (1977) suggested that the exceptionally large UV peak represents a stable, sensitizing pigment, which indirectly isomerizes rhodopsin's chromophore by first absorbing the UV energy and by reradiating it at longer wavelengths (via fluorescence) where the probability of absorption by rhodopsin is greater. This appears to be a novel way for increasing a receptor's absolute sensitivity, albeit at the expense of spectral discrimination.

(b) The cones of birds and reptiles often contain brilliantly colored oil droplets, 3 to 6 μm in diameter, within their ellipsoid. Because light must pass through these ellipsoids on its way to the outer segments, the oil droplets act as color filters, just as colored spectacles would if placed before an eye. Depending on the type of pigment they contain, the droplets are either clear, yellow, orange, or red. Usually, each is associated with the cone of a specific visual pigment. The oil droplets do not abolish the intrinsic three cone types; rather, they just shift the individual peak sensitivities 5 to 20 nm into the red and commensurately reduce the spectral bandwidth (Baylor and Hodgkin, 1973). Colored droplets act as short-wave cut-off filters and thereby may improve the eye's spectral resolution in the blue region of the spectrum. For example, orange droplets absorb 100% of any incident light whose wavelength is less than about 520 nm, whereas red droplets absorb completely below about 570 nm (Liebman and Granda, 1975). As shown in Figure 4.7, all visual pigments exhibit at least 20% of the maximal absorption at wavelengths less than their λ_{max}. In the absence of oil droplets, excitation of a blue-absorbing cone by a 450-nm blue light cannot be more than five times more effective than that of a green-absorbing cone. But if the green-absorbing cone contains an orange oil droplet, which should absorb the incident blue light, preferential excitation of the blue-absorbing cone would increase by an order of magnitude. Thus, oil droplets, in converse to the aforementioned sensitizing pigment, improve the eye's spectral resolution at the expense of absolute sensitivity.

5.2 Action spectra

As previously indicated, our knowledge of spectral sensitivities is based on two separate techniques, each measuring the wavelength variation of a different receptor component. Photometric techniques measure the pigments themselves and yield absorption spectra. Nonphotometric techniques measure the photoresponse and lead to action spectra. Because action spectra are pervasively used for the characterization of visual pigments (as illustrated in Figure 5.2*c*), this section will present the fundamental principles underlying action spectrum analysis and will discuss ways in which action spectra can differ from spectra obtained by photometric techniques.

An action spectrum is a plot of light intensity versus wavelength, where the ordinate refers to the intensity required to produce a given

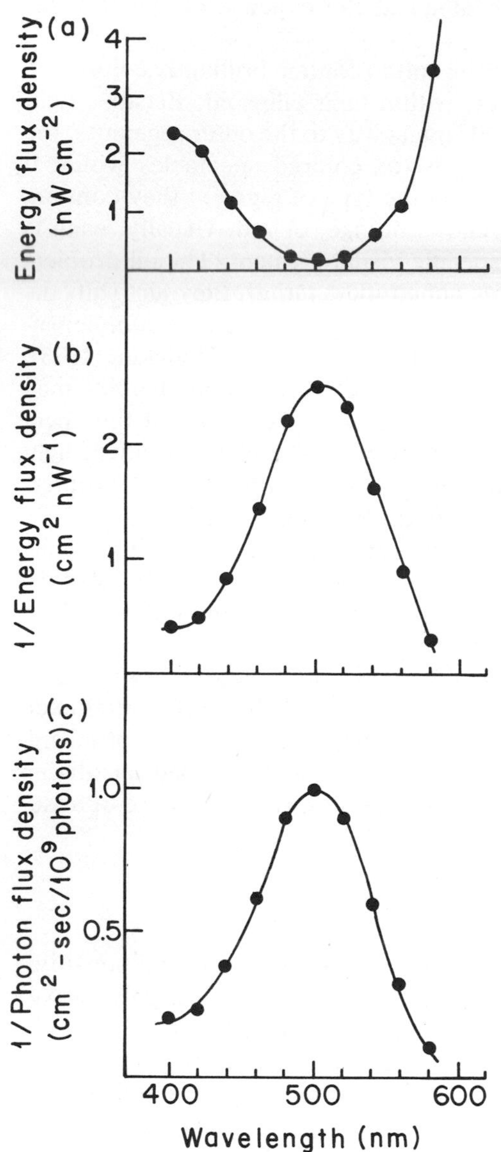

Figure 5.3. Action spectra plotted three ways using different ordinates. (*a*) Plot of incident energy flux density versus wavelength, where the ordinate is in units of nanowatts per square centimeter. (*b*) Plot of (incident energy flux density)$^{-1}$ versus wavelength, with the same units as in part (*a*). (*c*) Plot of (incident photon flux density)$^{-1}$ versus wavelength, where photon flux density is in units of photons per square centimeter-second. The

criterion response. Its aim is to characterize (by spectral shape and spectral location) the pigment(s) giving rise to the photoresponse. The nature of the monitored response is not crucial and is determined mainly by the type of experiment being performed. Electrophysiologists choose membrane potential excursions or response latencies, and psychophysicists depend on reproducible sensations. The spectral form of the action spectrum is entirely independent of the response measure chosen, provided that the criterion response is nonsaturating. To ensure nonsaturation, criterion-response amplitudes are selected to be near the lower end of their dynamic range. Thus, electrophysiologists choose a criterion response that leads to, say, a 5-mV membrane potential change, whereas psychophysicists select the visual threshold as their reference. Because photoreceptors are quantum detectors, generating a signal in proportion to the rate at which they absorb photons, the use of a criterion response ensures that at all wavelengths the photoreceptor absorbs the same number of photons. To keep this number constant, the number of photons in the incident beam must vary with wavelength.

Figure 5.3 illustrates common ways to plot action spectra. Though normally only the incident beam's energy is measured, it should bc converted to incident photons because visual cells are quantum detectors. Because absorptance is the ratio of absorbed to incident photons, (Section 4.6), an action spectrum plotted in terms of (incident photons)$^{-1}$ is actually a plot of the following equation:

$$1/n_i = (1/n_a)\,(1 - 10^{-\epsilon c l}) \qquad (5.1)$$

where n_i is the number of incident photons and n_a the number of absorbed photons, which is a constant. If absorption is due only to a single visual pigment, a cell's action spectrum should be identical to the absorptance spectrum of its pigment, where "identical" here means the λ_{max} of the two spectra is the same and the spectral shapes

Figure 5.3 (*cont.*)
data points were based on intracellular recordings of dark-adapted toad red rods (Fain, 1976). The action spectrum was generated by measuring the intensity necessary for a criterion response of 1.7 mV with 9-msec flashes of monochromatic diffuse light, whose wavelength was varied. The experimentally obtained intensities are usually in units of watts and should be converted to photons, as was done in (*c*), to reflect accurately the receptor's absorptance spectrum. For the cited experiment, the criterion response required a test flash that delivered about 10^7 photons cm^{-2} at 502 nm, equivalent to about three incident photons per rod. (After Rodieck, 1973.)

are superimposable (their absolute values will always differ by an undetermined constant).

Before an action spectrum can be attributed to a particular visual pigment, interfering pigments located either in front of the photoreceptor or even in the photoreceptor itself must be taken into account. Structures such as the dioptric apparatus, the screening pigments, the macular pigments, and the oil droplets of the ellipsoid themselves absorb light and can seriously distort action spectra. Additional consideration should also be given to receptor–receptor interactions. If coupling exists between cells with different visual pigments, the measured action spectrum will show a combined effect. This is the case for many, albeit not all, green and UV receptors in the honeybee eye. When these cells are electrically coupled to each other, the action spectrum of a UV cell, for example, will have a primary λ_{max} that is red shifted by as much as 30 nm and will also show a secondary maximum at 540 nm near the primary peak of the green receptors (Menzel and Blakers, 1976).

Even if interactions between unlike receptors are absent and the effects of interfering pigments can be corrected, cellular action spectra may not exactly match the pigment absorptance spectra. For example, this happens for human rods. Their action spectrum, measured psychophysically by the threshold criterion is significantly narrower than the predicted absorptance spectrum (Figure 5.4). The latter's prediction was based on the absorbance of the pigment (as measured by microspectrophotometry, with the measuring beam passing transversely through a single isolated outer segment) and on the assumption that in an intact eye light's path length through the outer segment is equal to that organelle's anatomical length. Recalling that absorptance spectra broaden with increasing path length (Section 4.6), the assumed path length in Figure 5.4 was overestimated because it generated a broader curve. Given the experimental errors, the effective path length of rods must be less by at least a factor of two to four. This could occur either because light obliquely traverses the outer segment, so that its path length is less than the organelle's anatomical length or because the effectiveness of photoreceptor excitation is greater in the basal region of the outer segment. Though no direct experimental proof exists for the second alternative, it is known that excitation effectiveness can vary by as much as a factor of two between proximal and distal regions in toad rod outer segments (Baylor et al., 1979*b*). Experimental evidence in favor of the first alternative is also lacking, but if it were correct, then the reasons for the existence of long outer segments (in some deep-sea fish, they reach lengths of 200 μm; Munk, 1966) and the reasons for the pupillary orientation of photoreceptors (to be discussed in Section 5.3.3) would be unclear.

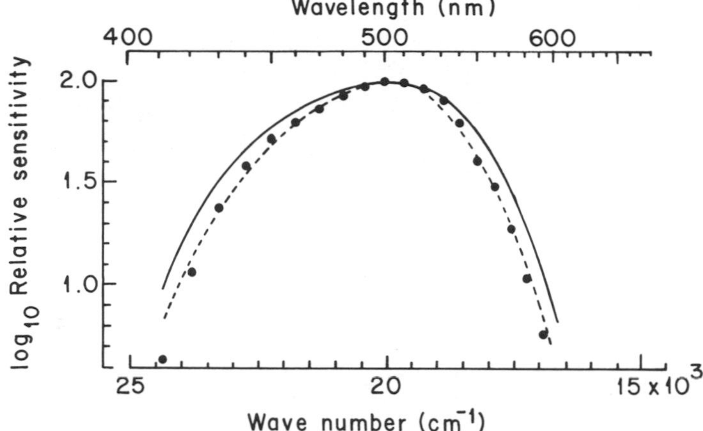

Figure 5.4. Comparison between the absorptance spectrum of human rods (solid and dashed lines) and the action spectrum of scotopic vision (●). The absorptance spectrum shown by the solid line was calculated from microspectrophotometric data, assuming that light's path length l through the outer segment is 26 μm, which is the anatomical length of the organelle. The dashed curve represents the absorptance spectrum limit as light's path length approaches zero ($l \rightarrow 0$ μm). See text for an interpretation of the results. (After Bowmaker and Dartnall, 1980.)

5.3 Polarization detection

In analogy to color vision, the underlying mechanism that makes polarization detection possible is ultimately based on the absorption properties of rhodopsin. Polarization detection, however, does not require different classes of pigment, each with a different λ_{max}. Rather it depends on the preferential alignment of large numbers of rhodopsin molecules within a receptor. How such an alignment leads to polarization detection will be described next.

5.3.1 Linear dichroism

For any absorbing molecule, the transition moment vector giving rise to a specific absorption band has a fixed orientation with respect to the molecule's three-dimensional structure. For example, the α-band transition moment for the chromophore is roughly parallel to its polyene chain (see Section 4.5). Light absorption by an individual molecule is maximal when the electric field vector **E** of the incident light is parallel to the transition moment, and absorption is minimal

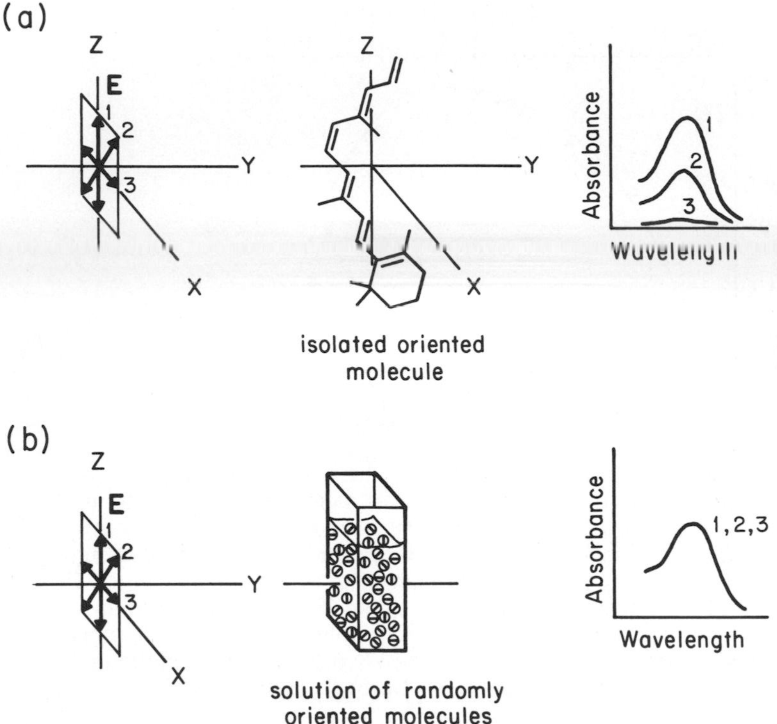

Figure 5.5. Dependence of light absorption on the relative orientation between the transition moment vector of a pigment molecule and the **E**-vector of a linearly polarized light. (*a*) Absorption by a single fixed molecule, when illuminated with polarized light, whose **E**-vector assumes any one of the three given orientations. The transition moment vector's exact orientation to the retinal's structure is unknown and is shown here parallel to the *z*-axis. (*b*) Absorption by a homogeneous solution of visual pigments, when illuminated with polarized light, whose **E**-vector assumes any one of the three given orientations. In the solution, each circle represents a single rhodopsin molecule, with a bar denoting the chromophore's transition moment vector.

when the **E**-vector is perpendicular to it (Figure 5.5). At other orientations, absorption is intermediate. Similar considerations apply for an ensemble of molecules, except that the average orientation of the ensemble must then be taken into account. If the molecules are randomly oriented, as in a solution, all orientations of the transition moments will occur with equal probability. This is because in a solution the thermal energy of the molecules causes them to tumble and to diffuse in all directions. At any given instant, just as many transition moments will be aligned along one direction as along any other, so that the sum of individual transition moments will be the same along any direction. Thus, linearly polarized light traveling along, say, the *z*-axis (see Figure 5.5 *b*) will be equally absorbed, irrespective of the direction of its **E**-vector. For preferential absorption to occur, the transition moments must be partially aligned; the direction of alignment will determine the direction in which the electric field vector must point for maximal absorption. If in Figure 5.5 all the molecules in the solution were somehow aligned with the *x*-axis, then maximal absorption would occur with the **E**-vector pointing along the *x*-axis, and minimal absorption, with it aligned to the *y*-axis. Such a preferential orientation within receptors is a prerequisite for polarization detection.

Unequal absorption of linearly polarized light about two mutually perpendicular axes is called *linear dichroism*. The larger absorption value divided by the smaller one is termed the *dichroic ratio* and is a direct function of the anisotropy of an ensemble of molecules. From its experimentally determined value, the average transition moment orientation can be derived.

Photoreceptor outer segments and rhabdoms are dichroic structures (see Figure 5.6, and for a recent review of the vertebrate literature, see Harosi, 1981). When outer segments are illuminated from the side, preferential absorption occurs when the electric field vector is parallel to the plane of the disks, implying that the transition moment vectors are partially aligned in that plane. Their degree of alignment, calculated from the measured dichroic ratio of 4 to 5 (Harosi and MacNichol, 1974*a*), indicates that the transition moments of the chromophores are tilted, on the average, about 17° from the plane of the membrane (Liebman, 1962; Harosi and Malerba, 1975). However, within the plane of the disk membrane, the chromophores are randomly oriented, so that dichroism is not observed for polarized light traveling axially along the outer segment's length (Figure 5.6*b*).

For invertebrate rhabdomeres, the axis of preferential absorption is parallel to the microvillar axis (Figure 5.6). Measured values for the dichroic ratio vary between 1 and 2 in fly receptors (Langer and Thorell, 1966), between 2 and 3 for isolated crayfish rhabdoms (Goldsmith, 1975), and may be as large as 6 in squid (Hagins, 1972). A ratio of about 1.7 can be solely attributed to the characteristic tubular structure of the microvilli because such a value would be obtained if vertebrate disk membranes were rolled into cylindrical shapes (see the review by Snyder, 1979). Because the dichroic ratio of crayfish rhabdoms is higher than the theoretical value of 1.7, the chromophore in crayfish must be partially aligned along the microvillar axis. Calcula-

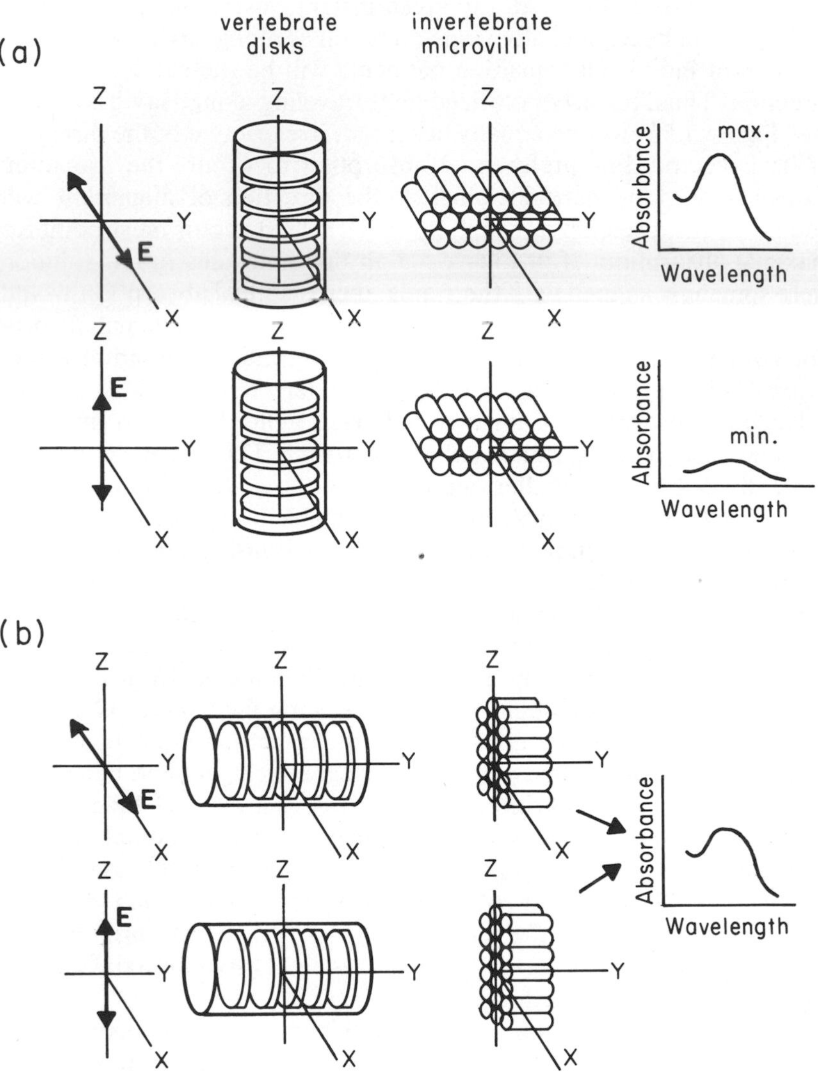

Figure 5.6. Differential absorption of linearly polarized light by vertebrate outer segments and rhabdomeric microvilli. (*a*) Light transversely incident to the long axis of the outer segments and of the microvilli. Maximal absorption occurs whenever the **E**-vector is parallel to the disk surface and to the microvillar axis. Though not indicated as such in this figure, the relative values for maximal and minimal absorptions are not the same for disks and microvilli; see text. (*b*) Light axially incident along the outer segment and the microvilli. Absorption is the same for all possible **E**-vector orientations.

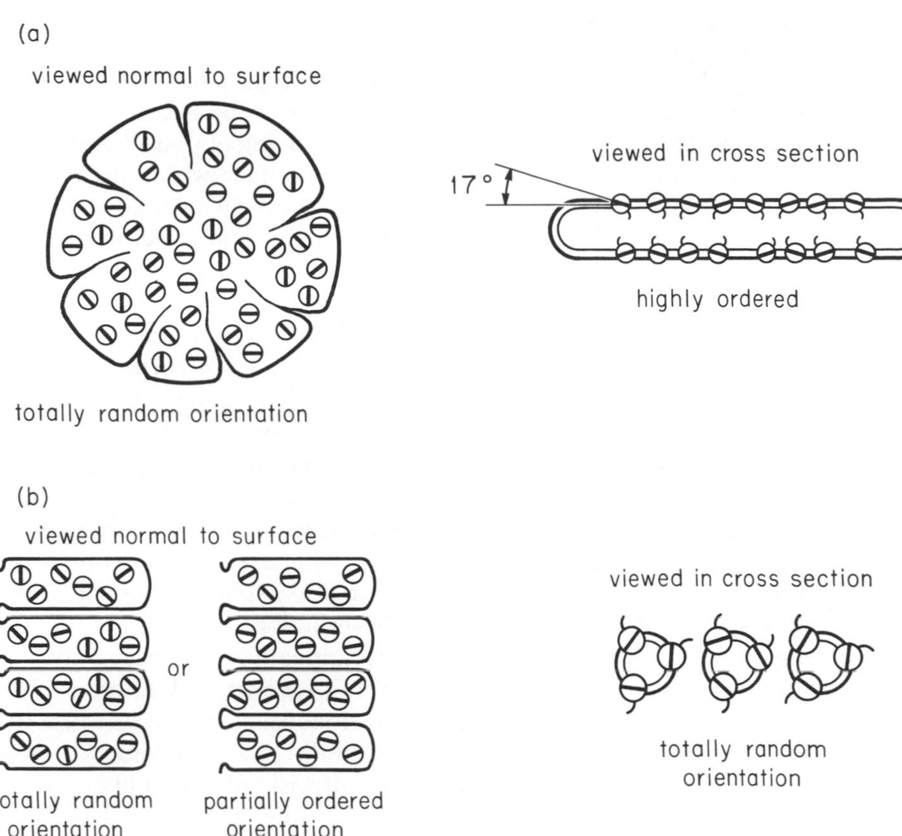

Figure 5.7. Summary of chromopore orientations within photoreceptor membranes: (*a*) ciliary disks; (*b*) rhabdomeric microvilli. Each circle represents a single rhodopsin molecule, with the bar denoting the chromophore's transition moment vector. The comma affixed to each circle stands for rhodopsin's sugar groups, which face either the extracellular or intradiskal solutions. For the cross-sectional views, note that individual chromophores are always highly oriented with respect to the membrane. However, because microvilli are circular in cross section, the chromophores assume all possible orientations within the plane of the cross section. It is for this reason that rhodopsins are identified as totally random in the cross-sectional view of (*b*).

tions indicate that their average transition moment vectors cannot make an angle greater than about 50° with the microvillar axis (Goldsmith and Wehner, 1977). Figure 5.7 summarizes chromophore orientation within ciliary disks and rhabdomeric microvilli.

5.3.2 Rhodopsin diffusion in the membrane

The highly fluid nature of the hydrophobic phase of membranes is by now well established (see the review by Edidin, 1974). The fluid state of membranes permits free intermixing of phospholipids and membrane proteins, as they translationally diffuse within the plane of the membrane. Such movements do not always occur, however, because sometimes they are hindered by cytoplasmic structures.

The fluid state of vertebrate receptor membranes was first demonstrated by Brown (1972) and Cone (1972) with their discovery that rhodopsin molecules freely spin about an axis normal to the disk surface. Because the spinning results from random Brownian movement caused by intermolecular collisions, it is known as *rotational diffusion*. The experimentally observed rotational rates imply that the lipid phase of disk membranes is about 100 times more viscous than water, comparable to the viscosity of olive oil and to most other biological membranes. The rotational diffusion of rhodopsin explains why outer segments are not dichroic with axial illumination – the chromophore and its transition moment can assume all possible orientations within the plane of the disk. Observations by later investigators demonstrated that, besides diffusing rotationally, rhodopsin could also diffuse laterally (Poo and Cone, 1974; Liebman and Entine, 1974). Lateral diffusion rates are such that if rhodopsins on one side of a frog disk are bleached, intermixing of the unbleached and bleached molecules is complete within 20 to 30 sec. Surprisingly, attempts to detect rotational and lateral diffusion of invertebrate rhodopsins have been unsuccessful in crayfish and squid, the only invertebrates in which it has been attempted (Goldsmith and Wehner, 1977; Foster, 1980), even though the lipid phase of squid microvilli is relatively fluid.

5.3.3 Polarization detection in selected organisms

It is the dichroic nature of the pigment-containing membranes that ultimately determines whether or not a visual system is capable of polarization detection. As determined by microscopy (Laties, 1969; Laties and Enoch, 1971; Baylor and Fettiplace, 1975; also see the review by Enoch, 1981) and X-ray diffraction (Webb, 1972), the axes of vertebrate outer segments all point to the front of the eye, with the axes intersecting each other somewhere near the center of the pupil. A consequence of their orientation is that light preferentially propagates axially down the outer segment, with its electric field vector always perpendicular to the disk surface. Axial propagation is also aided by light funneling within the inner segments and by wave guiding within the outer segments (see the review by Enoch, 1963). As illustrated in

Figure 5.6, outer segments are not dichroic when illuminated axially and, hence, cannot preferentially absorb polarized light. This explains why, in general, vertebrates lack polarization sensitivity. An additional consequence of the dichroic nature of disks is that the pupillary orientation of the outer segment ensures maximal light absorption. Thus vertebrates appear to have sacrificed polarization detection in favor of photosensitivity.

The subcellular processes responsible for the pupillary alignment of outer segments are not that well understood. Apparently, alignment occurs because within the subretinal space the photoreceptors can tilt with respect to the surface of the retina. The receptors bend at the level of the external limiting membrane, keeping their inner and outer segments aligned with each other. Such receptor tilt is illustrated by the cells of Figure 3.1. Pupillary alignment, which in humans has long been considered as a possible explanation of the psychophysically determined Stiles–Crawford effect (see the reviews by Rodieck, 1973, and Enoch, 1981), is apparently controlled by an active light-dependent process. Outer segment axes misalign whenever their receptors are kept in darkness for extended periods (Webb, 1977; Enoch et al., 1979).

The preceding considerations predict that for polarization detection to exist in vertebrates, the plane of the disks should not be perpendicular to the outer segment axis. This, in fact, occurs in anchovy cones (Fineran and Nicol, 1976), as is illustrated in Figure 5.8. The unique orientation of the disks and their mutual perpendicularity within adjacent cells suggest that the eyes of anchovies are polarization-sensitive.

All invertebrates with compound- or cephalopod-type eyes are potentially capable of polarization detection. As seen in Chapter 2, the receptor microvilli in these eyes are invariably oriented perpendicular to the visual axis and hence to the direction of incident light. As discussed in the previous section, this is the required orientation for preferential excitation by polarized light. In studying the response of photoreceptors to polarized light, physiologists typically measure a quantity known as *polarization sensitivity,* which, in analogy with the dichroic ratio, is defined as the ratio of the two light intensities that are needed to elicit a criterion response when the receptor is illuminated with linearly polarized light parallel and perpendicular to the axis of preferential absorption. (The use of "polarization sensitivity" for receptors is unfortunate because it incorrectly implies that individual cells are polarization discriminators. This issue will be reconsidered at the end of this section.) Just as action spectra do not always match absorptance spectra, so do polarization sensitivities poorly correlate with microvillar dichroic ratios. For example, polarization sensitivity can be as low as 1 to 1.3 in the fly (Scholes, 1969) and as large as 10 in the crayfish (Shaw, 1969) and the honeybee (Labhart, 1980).

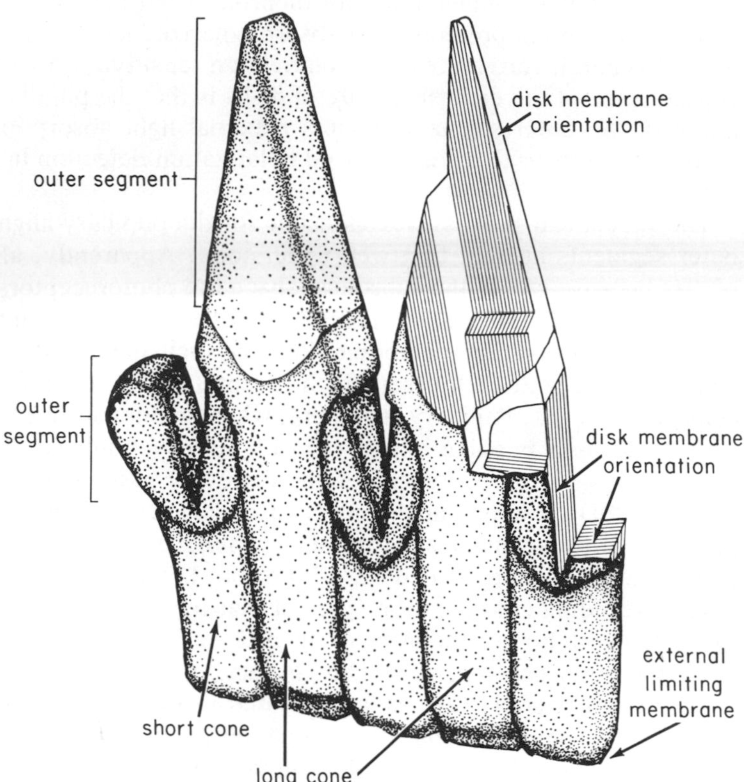

Figure 5.8. The cones of anchovies, showing their three-dimensional morphology distal to the external limiting membrane. Note that the outer segment of the short cone is divided into two equal lobes; it is "bifid." The cutaway areas on the right demonstrate the orientation of the disks and the manner in which the outer segment of the short cone presses into the ellipsoid of the long cone. (After Fineran and Nicol, 1978.)

Several factors can decrease a receptor's polarization sensitivity from the known dichroic ratio of its microvillus: (a) axially long rhabdomeres that absorb nearly the same percentage of light intensity for the two mutually perpendicular orientations, i.e., a large absorbance (Shaw, 1969); (b) variable microvillar orientations within a given receptor (Menzel, 1975); and (c) electrical coupling between retinular cells.

To illustrate how factor (b) affects polarization sensitivity, consider the worker honeybee, the classic example for a polarization-sensitive organism. In most of its ommatidia, rhabdoms are twisted about the ommatidial axis like the skeins of a rope (Figure 5.9). Though the villi

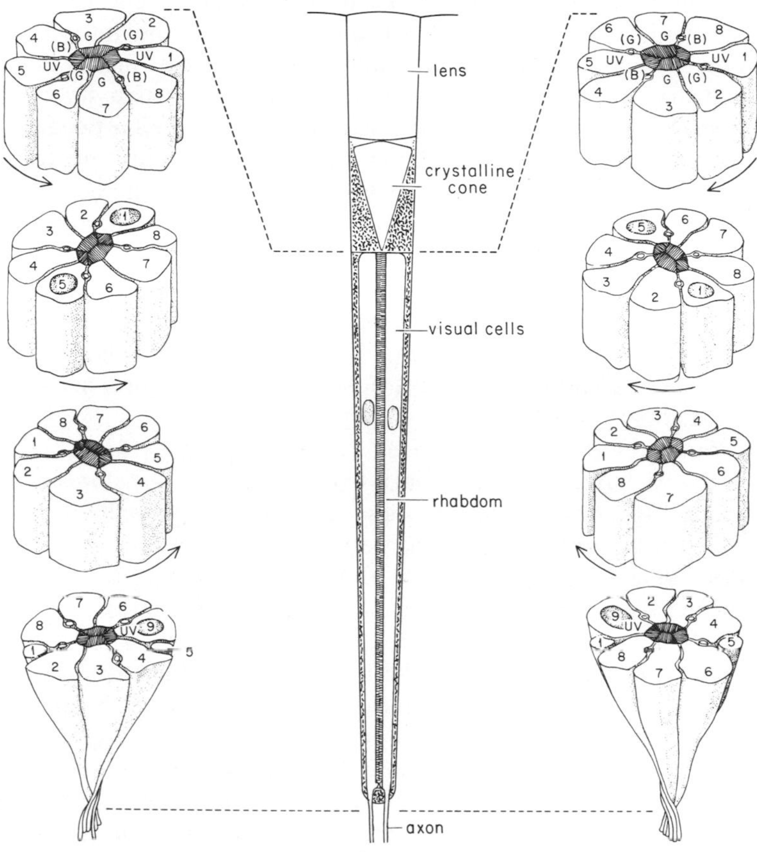

Figure 5.9. The morphology of the twisting, fused rhabdoms of the honeybee, characteristic over most of its compound eye. Each ommatidium contains nine retinular cells, which are numbered according to the convention of Menzel and Blakers (1976). The first eight cells are long; the ninth is short and is proximally located near the basement membrane. All nine cells are twisted. In half of the bee's ommatidia, the twist is clockwise, in the remainder, anticlockwise. The two kinds of ommatidia appear to be randomly distributed. Cells 1–8 are twisted 180° about the ommatidial axis, and cell 9 is twisted only 40° because of its shorter length. Of all the receptors, only cell 9 is polarization-sensitive. The wavelength region to which specific receptors are maximally sensitive is identified, with tentative assignations in parentheses. Respective λ_{max} values are: 360 nm for the ultraviolet cell (UV); 440 nm for the blue cell (B), and 540 nm for the green cell (G). (Illustration after Wehner, 1976; spectral data from Menzel and Blakers, 1976.)

remain perpendicular to the visual axis, the net effect of their variable orientations is to degrade for the whole cell the intrinsic dichroic property of the individual microvilli. Nevertheless, one of the retinular cells (cell 9) has a relatively large polarization sensitivity because the twisting of its short rhabdoms is more limited, being twisted only 40° rather than the 180° observed in the other cells. This apparently is the only cell the honeybee can employ for polarization detection within its lateral and ventral visual field. On the other hand, for navigation purposes, a distinct group of 140 ommatidia at the eye's dorsal rim are utilized. The facets at the dorsal rim are directed at the sky's zenith whenever an insect assumes a normal flying posture. The rhabdoms in these ommatidia do not twist (Wehner et al., 1975) and, as might be expected, some of these cells possess a "polarization sensitivity," of 10 (Labhart, 1980).

Several factors can enhance a receptor's "polarization sensitivity." These include: (a) preferential absorption by the rhabdoms of a preceding cell whenever two or more receptors line up axially in an ommatidium, (b) "optical coupling" between the receptors of a fused rhabdom, where light transmission along any specific rhabdomere depends on the absorption properties of all the rhabdomeres (Snyder et al., 1973), and (c) synaptic inhibition between receptors. Of the three factors, the last appears to be the most plausible explanation for the exceptionally large sensitivities reported for crayfish and honeybee eyes. Such inhibitory interactions are known to be responsible for the related process of contrast enhancement, which was initially discovered in *Limulus* photoreceptors and which has been observed in most other visual systems. However, its role in polarization detection has not yet been thoroughly investigated.

Though electrophysiologists attribute a certain "polarization sensitivity" value to a receptor, it should be emphasized that single receptors are not polarization detectors, just as they are not color detectors. Being quantum detectors, receptors cannot simultaneously transmit information about intensity and degree of polarization. *To detect light's polarization, an organism requires at least two classes of photoreceptors, each having a different axis of preferential excitation by polarized light.* In addition, its brain must be able to distinguish between the differential excitation of the two classes.

5.4 Summary

Though individual visual cells can preferentially respond to specific wavelengths or **E**-vector orientations, photoreceptors are not discriminators of these parameters. Being quantum detectors, they are incapable of simultaneously providing information on light intensity, polarization, and wavelength. To detect light's spectral composition or degree of polarization, visual systems must measure the output discrepancy from several types of receptors, each of which is equally sensitive to intensity yet differentially responsive to either of the other two parameters.

6 The visual cycle of rhodopsin

Having considered spatial resolution, color vision, and polarization detection in the previous chapters, only the detection of intensity remains to be discussed in terms of its underlying mechanism. Intensity detection, which requires receptor signal generation in response to absorbed photons, basically represents the primary function of photoreceptors. Spatial resolution, color vision, and polarization detection are possible mainly because neighboring receptors absorb photons at different rates.

The molecular events that make intensity detection possible will be the focus for the remainder of this book. This chapter will consider the effects of photon absorption on rhodopsin, and Chapters 7–12 will examine its effect on subsequent molecular processes.

As Boll and Kühne demonstrated in the 1870s, rhodopsin is unstable in the presence of light. When it absorbs a photon, the molecule spontaneously and rapidly progresses through a sequence of transient states, without the need of enzymatic or metabolic energy. Irrespective of the identity of the organism, the ultimate effect of these reactions is to yield products that are stable with time. With solubilized pigments, the products are indeed very stable. Within photoreceptors, however, the end products gradually disappear as they are recycled for resynthesis of the original pigment. In contrast to the cascade of spontaneous reactions, the regenerative reactions are energy-consuming. The entire process through which the visual pigment proceeds, from photoactivation to regeneration, has been termed the *visual cycle* (Wald, 1935).

6.1 The three types of light-induced transitions

Although the intermediates of the visual cycle have been primarily characterized in terms of their spectral properties, it is important to realize that spectral shifts are not the only consequence of photon absorption. The cascade of light-induced conformational changes, which involve the tertiary and possibly the secondary structure of rhodopsin, give rise to three types of concurrent transitions:

1. the aforementioned spectral shifts,
2. a sequence of charge displacements within the protein chain itself, and
3. a transformation into a biochemically "active state."

Of the three transitions, the last is of primary importance because it is responsible for initiating the biochemical dark reactions of phototransduction; it constitutes *rhodopsin's physiological function*. Though the mechanism whereby rhodopsin performs this function still remains obscure at this writing, enough biochemical evidence is available to suggest tentatively that animal rhodopsin behaves very similarly to hormone receptors and is unlike the proton-pumping bacteriorhodopsin of halophilic bacteria. (This aspect of rhodopsin's biochemistry will be extensively treated in Chapter 11). As far as the photoreceptor is concerned, the remaining intramolecular transitions, the spectral shifts, and the charge displacements are of little importance to transduction. It is ironic that our knowledge in these areas is so much more complete.

Just as spectrophotometric methods are needed to study rhodopsin's spectral intermediates, electrophysiological techniques are required to detect the aforementioned charge displacements of the molecule. The movement of these charges generate potentials, which were discovered by Brown and Murakami (1964) and which were named by them the *early receptor potential* (ERP), because these potentials temporally precede the photoreceptor's light response or receptor potential (which will be discussed in subsequent chapters.)

As Hagins and McGaughy (1967) showed for invertebrates and Cone (Cone, 1967; Cone and Cobbs, 1969) for vertebrates, there is a nearly one-to-one correspondence between these charge displacements and spectral transitions. Both obey the same kinetics. Such a correspondence holds as long as the chromophore and the protein remain attached to each other. Following the discussion of the visual cycle, the salient features and the generating mechanism of the ERP will be considered.

6.2 The visual cycle of vertebrates and invertebrates

Figures 6.1 and 6.2 summarize the visual cycle of typical and well-characterized vertebrate and invertebrate pigments: the rhodopsin ($R500_1$) of living rat and the solubilized UV-absorbing pigment ($R345_1$) of *Ascalaphus*, respectively. The intermediates of the cycle are so arranged that bathorhodopsin, the intermediate with the highest free energy, is located at the apex, and the stable reaction products with the

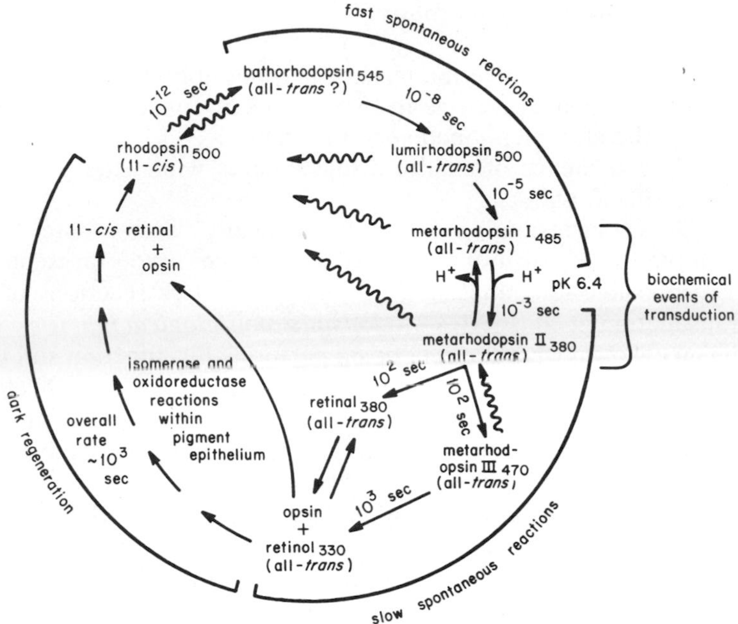

Figure 6.1. The visual cycle of rat rhodopsin. Photochemical reactions are denoted by wavy lines; dark reactions (either spontaneous or enzymatic) by straight lines. Each intermediate's λ_{max} appears as a subscript, with the conformation of its chromophore in parentheses. Metarhodopsins are usually abbreviated as "meta," with the appropriate Roman numeral following it. For a full description of the cycle, see text. Note, the decay of meta II can form either meta III or "retinal," the latter being a chromophore–protein complex that is spectrally indistinguishable from free retinal. Both meta III and "retinal" lead to the formation of opsin and all-*trans* retinol. The latter molecule, which freely moves between the receptor cell and the pigment epithelium, is oxidized and isomerized by energy consuming dark reactions to yield 11-*cis* retinal. It then spontaneously reacts with opsin, which did not move beyond the confines of its membrane, to regenerate rhodopsin. The cited rate constant for the formation of each spectral intermediate refers to physiological temperatures. The rate for the rhodopsin → bathorhodopsin transition was obtained for rhodopsin solutions, and the rates for the remainder of the bleaching cycle were obtained on excised rat retinas (Cone and Cobbs, 1969; Poo and Cone, unpublished observations). The identity of the individual reactions by which all-*trans* retinol is converted to 11-*cis* retinal has been left out; the time course for the overall process is from Yoshikami and Nöll (1979). The above cycle refers to the intact eye. For an isolated retina, devoid of its pigment epithelium, dark regeneration is absent. And if rhodopsin is solubilized, the kinetics of the spontaneous reactions are also altered.

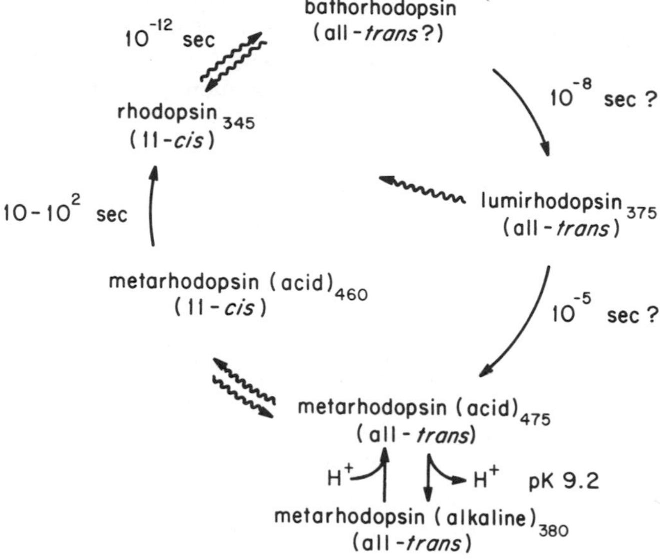

Figure 6.2. The visual cycle of the UV-absorbing pigment of *Ascalaphus*. As before, photochemical reactions are denoted by wavy lines and thermal reactions by straight lines. The rate constant for the $M_{460} \rightarrow R_{345}$ transition is from Hamdorf and Schwemer (1975). The compound eye of *Ascalaphus macaronius*, the owl fly, is of the superposition type. It consists of two anatomically distinct sections, the so-called frontal and lateral eyes, whose ommatidia differ in size but not in general structure (Schneider et al., 1978). Each ommatidium contains six large and two small retinula cells, the latter possibly being polarization-sensitive. The frontal eye is sensitive to ultraviolet light exclusively (Gogala, 1967), whereas the lateral eye also responds to blue-green light. This insect is active only in bright sunshine.

lowest free energy are on the bottom. Rhodopsin begins its journey through the cycle whenever the photochemical reaction converts it to bathorhodopsin. The cascade of subsequent spontaneous reactions is analogous to the spontaneous decay of unstable atoms or molecules to lower energy states.

Photostationary studies at low temperatures (Yoshizawa, 1972) indicate that yet another intermediate, hypsorhodopsin, may temporally precede bathorhodopsin. Hypsorhodopsin was omitted from the figures because its in vivo or in situ existence has not yet been confirmed.

The vertebrate and invertebrate cycles share several properties: both consist of the aforementioned spontaneous and regenerative reactions and both share the same initial spectral intermediates. The shared intermediates (batho-, lumi-, and metarhodopsins) comprise the fast reactions of the spontaneous cascade. They occur on a time scale of milliseconds. The time courses of subsequent intermediates, which take minutes or even hours, are characteristically found only within vertebrates. Note that *photolysis*, the splitting of the visual pigment into free chromophore and opsin, occurs only within vertebrates. Because these separated end products are colorless, the complete set of spontaneous reactions for vertebrates is referred to as the *bleaching sequence*. Though most of our understanding about the spontaneous thermal reactions was obtained with solubilized pigments, early receptor potential measurements with live rats (Cone and Cobbs, 1969) and photometric studies with isolated frog retinas (Baumann, 1972, 1976; Cone, 1972) have clearly confirmed that, starting with the decay of bathorhodopsin, the same set of reactions occurs within the receptors at physiological temperatures. Bacteriorhodopsin's (R568) visual cycle is very similar to that of animal rhodopsin in that it also cascades through a sequence of thermal reactions, its important difference being that the thermal reactions terminate with the regeneration of the parent pigment (for its cycle, see Honig, 1978).

The conformational transformations within the molecule as it proceeds through the spectral intermediates need not and probably do not represent major structural changes. For example, the known spectral transitions between the oxy and the deoxy forms of hemoglobin are due to very small displacements between subunits, whose secondary and tertiary structures remain unaltered. Similarly, circular dichroism measurements on disk membranes indicate no light-induced changes in rhodopsin's secondary structure when the pigments are within their native membrane (Shichi, 1971). Even fixation with gluteraldehyde, a cross-linking agent that binds the pigments into an unextractable matrix, does not eliminate or arrest the spontaneous reactions in frogs and squids (Brown, 1972; Hagins and McGaughy, 1967). The observation with fixatives, however, should not be taken as conclusive proof, because spectral properties reflect only the microenvironment surrounding the chromophore. For example, the proteolysis of rhodopsin with papain, which dissociates the molecule into a small water-soluble component and two equally large membrane-associated fragments, has no effect on either rhodopsin's absorption spectrum or on the extent of its regenerability (Fung and Hubbell, 1978*a*).

6.3 Bathorhodopsin formation

Bathorhodopsin represents the photoactivated state of the visual pigment. The probability of its formation, following photon absorption by rhodopsin, is given by the quantum efficiency of photoactivation and is about 0.7 (see Section 4.7). Once it is formed, bathorhodopsin cannot revert back to rhodopsin in the dark but must spontaneously decay through a series of intermediates. The spontaneous reactions, however, can be arrested and bathorhodopsin can be stabilized if temperatures are decreased to those of liquid nitrogen. The activation energy needed for bathorhodopsin's formation is at least 45 kcal $mole^{-1}$ (Cooper, 1979). This energy barrier can be readily crossed by photon absorption, because the energy content of a mole of photons at 500 nm is 57 kcal. In this reaction, about 60% of the photon's energy is transferred to and stored in bathorhodopsin. As indicated in Figure 6.1, the kinetics of bathorhodopsin formation and decay are extremely fast at physiological temperatures: respective half-times are a few picoseconds and 10 nsec.

On the structural level, light's effect on the chromophore is still unknown. Hubbard and Kropf (1958) suggested that light converts the 11-*cis* chromophore to an all-*trans* state. Their suggestion was based partly on the finding that denaturation of unbleached rhodopsin with strongly alkaline solutions decomposes the pigment to opsin plus 11-*cis* retinal, whereas similar denaturation of lumi- or metarhodopsin releases the chromophore as all-*trans* retinal. The same results were later obtained with bathorhodopsin, which was formed at liquid-nitrogen temperatures and subsequently denatured at higher temperatures (Yoshizawa and Wald, 1963). Thus, it was concluded that: (1) the state of the chromophore in bathorhodopsin is all-*trans* and, as a result, (2) the rhodopsin → bathorhodopsin transition represents an isomerization reaction.

The all-*trans* nature of bathorhodopsin's chromophore has been seriously challenged. The first experimental data inconsistent with the theory was obtained with chicken iodopsin. When bathoiodopsin was formed at −195°C and was subsequently warmed to −140°C in the dark, iodopsin was spontaneously regenerated (Hubbard et al., 1965). (Under physiological temperatures, however, reversion to iodopsin is as unfavored as for other visual pigments). Because isomerization reactions require much larger energies than are available from thermal energy (even at room temperature), the iodopsin → bathoiodopsin → iodopsin transitions could not have occurred solely by isomerization. Studies performed with cattle rhodopsin using ultrafast spectroscopy (Peters et al., 1977) and Raman spectroscopy (Oseroff and Callender, 1974; Lewis, 1978*a*) have raised further doubts. Peters and co-workers believe that the primary transition represents proton translocation between opsin and the chromophore, whereas Lewis proposes that it represents both proton translocation and torsional movement in the polyene chain. Though the temporal and causal relationship of proton displacement and isomerization remains to be settled, it is now generally agreed that the conformation of the chromophore in bathorhodopsin is at least partially, if not completely, all-*trans* (see the review by Birge, 1981). Irrespective of the intermediate at which the complete all-*trans* isomer is finally formed, Hubbard and Kropf's initial concept is still correct – light eventually leads to isomerization, or as reiterated so often, the "action of light in vision is to isomerize the chromophore of a visual pigment from the 11-*cis* to the all-*trans* configuration. Everything else that happens – chemically, physiologically, indeed psychologically – represents 'dark' consequences of this one light reaction" (Wald, 1968, p. 234).

6.4 Meta I → meta II transition

In contrast to the reactions preceding it, meta I → meta II is a reversible dark reaction that depends on the solution pH. A pH exceeding 6.4 favors meta II formation for rat rhodopsin. The acid and alkaline metarhodopsins of invertebrates are analogous to meta I and meta II of vertebrates. The p*K* of these dark reactions can be quite variable, ranging from 6.4 to 9.1. The formation of meta II is accompanied by a net uptake of one proton in both rhodopsin solutions (Matthews et al., 1963) and photoreceptor membranes (Falk and Fatt, 1966). Because this represents net movement, i.e., the difference between protons released and protons bound, the actual number of protons involved in the reaction is unknown. That at least a single proton per rhodopsin should have been released during the reaction is suggested by the blue-shifted λ_{max} of meta II. Deprotonation of the Schiff's base should cause such a spectral shift.

6.5 Slow spontaneous reactions

The actual pathway for the slow spontaneous reactions is not yet firmly established. First, it is not clear whether photoactivated rhodopsin passes through all the intermediates of Figure 6.1 when it is photoactivated at slow rates or in small amounts. This is because in almost all studies investigators photoactivate large amounts of pigment to be able to resolve the individual, spectrally overlapping intermediates. Azuma et al. (1977) have presented evidence suggesting that as long as flashes bleach less than about 2% of the initial pigment, rhodopsin within isolated retinas does not decay beyond meta II because it is quickly regenerated from that intermediate. According to their view, brighter intensities create so much meta II that they overwhelm the regenerating process, causing meta II to spill over into the routes that lead to photolysis. Further research is definitely needed to clarify this aspect of photochemistry.

Although it is now generally agreed that, following exhaustive bleaches, meta II must decay by two parallel paths, the convergence point of these routes has not yet been definitely settled. They may either converge at the retinol state, as illustrated in Figure 6.1 (Cone and Cobbs, 1969), or at "retinal" (Baumann, 1972). The former scheme appears to be equally applicable for all pigments for which in situ kinetics have been measured, including human, rat, frog, and skate rhodopsin (Ernst et al., 1978).

The preferential pathway and the kinetics of meta II decay apparently vary greatly among species. Almost 75% of human rhodopsin ($R498_1$) passes through meta III, whereas in carp, porphyropsin ($R525_2$) bleaches via "retinal" (Donner et al., 1974). Human and frog rhodopsins bleach much more slowly than other pigments. The rate constants appear to be several orders of magnitude greater for gecko pigments ($R521_1$) (Bowmaker, 1973) and about five times greater for the cone pigments of goldfish (Harosi and MacNichol, 1974*b*). The kinetics of the slow spontaneous reactions in the human eye are illustrated in Figure 6.3. As Figures 6.1 and 6.3 indicate, under physiological conditions, meta II is formed within a millisecond and decays very slowly, with a half-time of 100 sec. As will be discussed in the next chapter, the light-induced voltage response of photoreceptors is on the order of seconds. This means that if the meta II lifetime is independent of bleaching intensity, the visual pigment remains in the meta II state throughout most, if not the entire, photoreceptor response.

Because aldehydes are highly reactive, retinal is probably never free in the retina. The so-called "retinal" formed from meta II most likely represents a loosely and nonspecifically bound chromophore. Retinol, however, can freely exist, and because it is hydrophobic, it partitions into the lipid phase of the membrane with its polyene chain parallel to the fatty acids and its hydroxyl group at the membrane–water interface. To migrate from cell to cell across aqueous domains, retinal and its derivatives depend on specific transport proteins, which possess hydrophobic pockets into which the molecules readily partition. Such binding proteins, specific either for retinol or for 11-*cis* retinal, have been isolated from extracts of bovine retinas (Saari and Futterman, 1976; Futterman et al., 1977).

6.6 Photoconversion among isomers

Hubbard and Kropf (1958) discovered that when the initial spectral intermediates of the bleaching cycle absorb a photon, they can

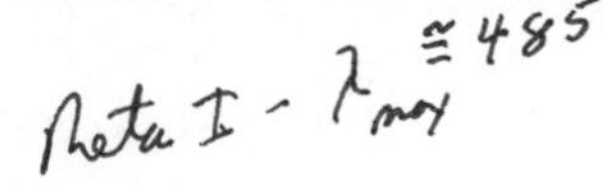

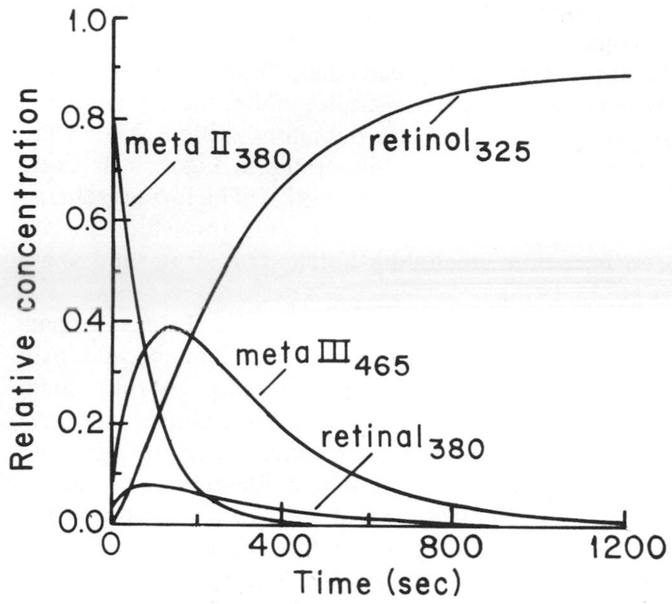

Figure 6.3. Time course for the buildup and decay of spectral intermediates during the slow spontaneous reactions of rhodopsin ($R498_1$) as measured within the isolated human retina. Each intermediate decays by a first-order process and is identified with a subscript, which refers to the pigment's λ_{max}. From the experimentally determined rate constants, the half-life of meta II is 58 sec; of meta III, 173 sec; and of "retinal," 23 sec. (After Baumann and Bender, 1973.)

either regenerate rhodopsin or, with a smaller probability, create a new pigment called isorhodopsin, whose chromophore is in the 9-*cis* form. Except for its blue-shifted λ_{max} (by 15 nm), isorhodopsin is similar to rhodopsin in most respects: it is thermally stable in the dark and can be photoactivated to yield the same sequence of spectral intermediates (Pratt, 1968).

The photochemical production of rhodopsin and isorhodopsin represents light-induced conversions among isomers. As mentioned in Chapter 4, the energy content of visible photons is much greater than the energy barriers separating the retinal isomers. Thus, photon absorption by any one isomer can easily convert it into another. The observed photoconversions provided the rationale for Hubbard and Kropf to suggest that isomerization occurred during the rhodopsin → bathorhodopsin transition. Isorhodopsin and regenerated rhodopsin formation require multiple, even-numbered photon absorptions by a molecule; the first absorption begins rhodopsin's cycle, and the second absorption converts an intermediate back to rhodopsin or isorhodopsin. When an isomer of free retinal is irradiated in solution, the result is a mixture of all-*trans*, 9-*cis*, 11-*cis*, and 13-*cis* isomers. However, when rhodopsin is irradiated, the 13-*cis* isomer is undetected, presumably because steric hindrance from opsin prevents its formation.

Although the initial observation of Hubbard and Kropf was performed with cattle rhodopsin extracts, photogeneration of both rhodopsin and isorhodopsin has also been observed within living vertebrates (Huddleston and Williams, 1977) and within some invertebrates (Hamdorf et al., 1973). Once isorhodopsin is formed within a receptor, it is not eliminated unless light photoactivates it, in which case it is as equally capable of generating an excitatory signal as rhodopsin (Pepperberg et al., 1976, 1978; Huddleston and Williams, 1977). The commonly observed photoisomerization pathways for vertebrate and invertebrate pigments are illustrated by the wavy lines in Figures 6.1 and 6.2. For the sake of simplicity, isorhodopsin formation was omitted from the figures.

Photogeneration has the important consequence that short-duration light flashes cannot exhaust a rhodopsin population, no matter how intense the flash energy. In fact, white light flashes that are less than 1 msec in duration cannot bleach more than about 50% of the pigment (Hagins, 1955, 1957; Williams, 1974).

To understand this phenomenon, one must consider the parameters involved in such photochemical reactions. The amount of rhodopsin photoregenerated from a specific intermediate by any stimulus can be simply expressed as

$$\begin{pmatrix}\text{rhodopsin molecules}\\ \text{photoregenerated}\\ \text{from intermediate}\end{pmatrix} = \begin{pmatrix}\text{quantum efficiency of}\\ \text{photoregeneration}\end{pmatrix} \times \begin{pmatrix}\text{absorbed photons/}\\ \text{molecule of intermediate}\end{pmatrix} \times (\text{molecules of intermediate}) \tag{6.1}$$

This equation holds only as long as photon absorption is restricted to the intermediate. As rhodopsin concentration increases, rhodopsin will begin to absorb, yielding additional spectral intermediates besides the initial one. With continuous light exposure, a steady state or photoequilibrium is achieved, with each molecule cycling back and forth among the various pigment states.

Quantum efficiencies in Equation (6.1) vary considerably among intermediates. For vertebrate pigments, the highest values (of about 0.3; Hubbard et al., 1965) belong to the reactions involving the batho-, lumi-, or meta I states. For some invertebrate rhodopsins, quantum efficiency of photoregeneration from meta may be as high as 0.7 (Hamdorf, 1979). Three factors determine how many photons can be absorbed by an intermediate: (1) the intermediate's absorption spectrum (the value of its ϵ at any wavelength), (2) the spectral composition of the incident light, and (3) the duration of the light stimulus relative to the lifetime of the intermediate.

The cited constraints provide the explanation of why intense flashes less than 1 msec cannot bleach vertebrate rhodopsin. The duration of such flashes is less than the sum of the lifetimes of the most easily reconvertible intermediates (batho-, lumi-, and meta I states). As a result, photoregeneration is maximal and bleaching minimal. As the flash duration becomes longer, photoregeneration is commensurately reduced and bleaching increased. Thus, steady illumination of vertebrate rhodopsin is always capable of completely bleaching the pigment and will do so if the stimulus is long enough and if enzymatic regeneration is absent. By contrast, steady illumination cannot exhaust invertebrate rhodopsin because invertebrate meta states are very stable with time and can readily photoregenerate their parent pigment.

Photoregeneration is an easy way to synthesize rhodopsin without the use of metabolic energy. As expected and as will be shortly discussed in greater detail, it plays a more important role for invertebrates than vertebrates.

6.7 Regeneration for vertebrates

In comparison with the bleaching sequence, the regeneration of vertebrate rhodopsin is rather poorly understood. Regeneration can occur either by enzymatic or by photochemical means. That the latter represents only a minor pathway can be demonstrated by comparing the photoactivation and photogeneration rates for human rhodopsin by a continuous source. A bright intensity that is commonly encountered by humans, say, in an office surrounding, may photoactivate about 5% rhodopsin min^{-1}, or 0.17% sec^{-1}. Using the principles previously discussed, one can calculate that the rates of photoregeneration from batho-, lumi-, and meta I states are more than a thousand times less than the rates of photoactivation. (This is primarily because their short lifetimes limits the number of photons they can absorb.) Because the quantum efficiency of regeneration from "retinal" is very low, meta II and III remain as the predominant intermediates from which rhodopsin could be photosynthesized. Given their lifetime (Figure 6.3), their relative extinction coefficients (Baumann, 1972), and the appropriate quantum efficiencies (Williams, 1968; Reuter, 1976), the calculated rate of photoregeneration from them is less than 6% of the rate of photoactivation. Thus over 94% of the bleached rhodopsin escapes the chance of photoregeneration and requires metabolic energy for resynthesis. Of course, photogeneration would be much more successful with brighter and shorter light flashes.

Although vertebrates rely almost solely on enzymatic regeneration, it is not yet clear from which spectral intermediates this (or these) reactions begin. Experiments in which visual pigments are completely bleached support the notion that enzymatic regeneration does not occur before the pigment is hydrolyzed to opsin and the free chromophore. As indicated previously, Azuma et al. (1977) presented evidence in opposition to this view. To regenerate rhodopsin from retinol, two reactions must happen (not necessarily in the order listed): (1) vitamin A must be isomerized to an 11-*cis* isomer via the enzyme isomerase and (2) it must be oxidized to the aldehyde via the NADPH-dependent oxidoreductase. It is not yet clear what fraction of these enzymatic activities occurs within the photoreceptors themselves and what fraction within the surrounding pigment epithelium. In this regard, variability among species is especially great.

That the pigment epithelium plays a major role in the regeneration of 11-*cis* retinal is overwhelming (Kühne, 1878). For instance, isolated retinas stripped of their pigment layer are unable to restore their visual pigment even when perfused with physiological saline solutions containing glucose and oxygen. Under the same conditions, the receptors maintain their light sensitivity for many hours (Sickel, 1965; Weinstein et al., 1967). Rhodopsin can be regenerated in such preparations only with an external application of 11-*cis* retinal (Pepperberg et al., 1978) or, in the case of frog, with the addition of 11-*cis* retinol (Yoshikami and Nöll, 1978). All-*trans* retinal and retinol applications have no effect. A more poignant observation in support of the role of pigment epithelium comes from the studies of Reuter et al., (1971) on the bullfrog. The rods of this retina contain either porphyropsin ($R522_2$) or rhodopsin ($R502_1$), with the two types of rods normally segregated into separate retinal regions. The corresponding regions of the epithelium store either vitamin A_1 or A_2. It was observed that the retina accepts whatever retinal the epithelium provides it. Thus, when two retinal regions are excised, bleached, and deliberately placed back onto each other's epithelial region, the pigment contents of the rods are exchanged; $R522_2$ for $R502_1$ and vice versa. The myriad pathways through which the chromophore can proceed on its way to 11-*cis* retinal formation are perhaps best characterized for the frog (Bridges, 1976).

The rate of pigment regeneration varies among pigments and among photoreceptors. For example, in vivo human cone pigments regenerate about four times faster than human rhodopsins (Rushton et al., 1955;

Rushton, 1957; also see the review by Rushton, 1972). Both processes follow a first-order exponential time course, with half-time being about 5 min for rods. It is not yet known which reaction in the visual cycle controls the observed rate. Although the rate of reaction between 11-*cis* retinal and cattle rod opsin in solutions is comparable to that of human rods in vivo (Hubbard and Wald, 1952), the analogous reaction rate for solubilized iodopsin is about 500 times faster (Wald et al., 1955). With photometric and ERP measurements, Yoshikami and Nöll (1979) observe that external applications of 11-*cis* retinal to the isolated rat retina regenerate rhodopsin within the plasma membrane about three times faster than the molecules within the disks. They also observe about the same absolute and relative rates in the eyes of anesthesized rats. Their observation suggests that, at least for rats, regeneration may be rate limited by translocation of the chromophore (in whatever state it is) across aqueous domains – extracellular space for cones and both extracellular and cytoplasmic space for rods.

6.8 Regeneration for invertebrates

Invertebrate rhodopsin can also be regenerated by parallel photochemical and enzymatic paths. In contrast with vertebrates, however, photoregeneration appears to be the predominant route. Direct evidence for this conclusion rests on studies performed with only two types of organisms – the octopus, *Eledone moschata* (Schwemer, 1969), and the owl fly, *Ascalaphus macaronius* (Hamdorf and Schwemer, 1975). These animals are well suited for photokinetic studies because their rhodopsins are spectrally well separated from their metarhodopsins. As a result, the formation and decay of either one of the states can be photometrically followed without any spectral interference from the other. The additional advantage with *Ascalaphus* is that its ommochrome screening pigments, which would ordinarily interfere with the optical measurements, can be easily removed. Figure 6.4*a* presents the absorption curves of R345 and its metarhodopsin M475 in *Ascalaphus*.

The enzymatic and photochemical regeneration processes of the isolated *Ascalaphus* eye are compared in Figure 6.5. Of the two reactions, photoregeneration is shown to be more than 300 times more efficient as measured by initial rates. Its rate could be even greater because the rate of photoregeneration is a linear function of light intensity (Hamdorf et al., 1973). A similar conclusion on the dominance of photoregeneration was also reported for the living retina of *Eledone,* albeit its dark regeneration was markedly greater than in *Ascalaphus* (Schwemer, 1969). An increased activity for the enzymatic

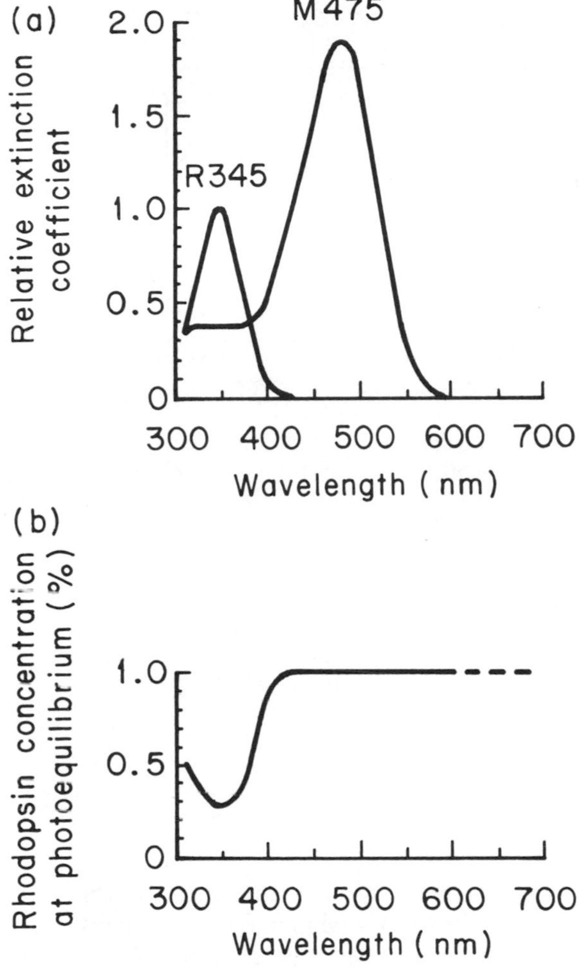

Figure 6.4. Spectral separation of rhodopsin and metarhodopsin in *Ascalaphus* and how it influences the percent rhodopsin concentration at photoequilibrium. (*a*) The relative extinction coefficients of R345 and M475, normalized to rhodopsin's maximal value. (*b*) The percentage of rhodopsin concentration at photoequilibrium as a function of the wavelength of incident monochromatic light. (After Hamdorf et al., 1973.)

process is not surprising because *Eledone* is mainly active in dim light. It would be interesting to know if chemical regeneration plays an even greater role in more nocturnal invertebrates. Unfortunately, direct photometric evidence is lacking.

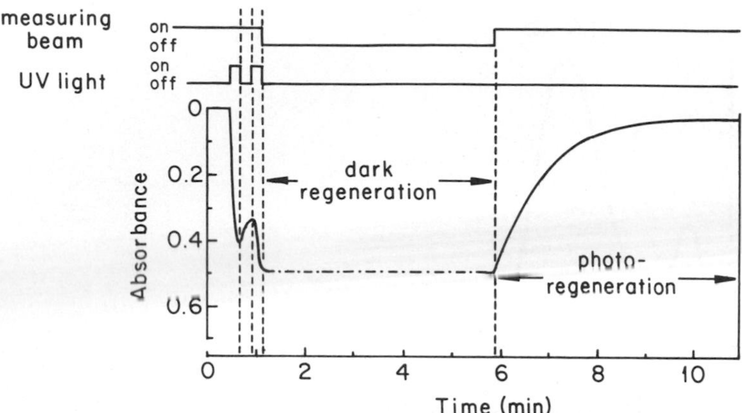

Figure 6.5. Rhodopsin (R345) regeneration within the isolated *Ascalaphus* eye by enzymatic and photochemical means. The eye's absorbance is monitored at 474 nm, a wavelength that is absorbed only by metarhodopsin. At the start, absorbance is minimal because all the pigment is in the R345 form. Ultraviolet irradiation converts rhodopsin to M475, thereby increasing absorbance. When UV irradiation is terminated the measuring beam photoconverts some of M475 back to R345 (between 0.6 and 0.9 min on time axis). Additional UV irradiation further increases the percentage concentration of M475. The measuring beam was turned off at 1.1 min so that only the dark regenerative reactions could proceed. When it was turned on again, at 5.9 min, initial absorbance was essentially the same as at 1.1 min, implying negligible dark regeneration. If the measuring beam is left on, it photoregenerates R345 with a half-time of about 1 min. (After Hamdorf and Schwemer, 1975.)

In those organisms where photoregeneration is the only, or the primary, means of rhodopsin synthesis, the visual pigments essentially exist as either rhodopsin or metarhodopsin. The other intermediates, of course, may also be present at certain times, but their concentration will be relatively low. The parameters determining photoconversion between the two stable states are given by Equation (6.1). If illumination is continuous, the states rapidly achieve photoequilibrium, with a final relative concentration being a function of the spectral composition of the incident light. Figure 6.4*b* illustrates the effects of continuous illumination on the pigment composition in *Ascalaphus*. Monochromatic lights with wavelengths above about 420 nm are absorbed only by M475, yielding a pigment population that is 100% rhodopsin. On the other hand, irradiation with shorter wavelengths, where the absorption spectra of R345 and M475 overlap, leads to a mixture of the two states. The relative concentration of rhodopsin and metarhodopsin at photoequilibrium is exactly the same as the ratio of the extinction coefficients at the irradiating wavelength. Thus, with a spectrally continuous light source, it is impossible to convert all the pigment to M475. The wide spectral separation of the two pigment states in *Ascalaphus* provides a very high rhodopsin concentration in the freely moving insect under natural light conditions. Sunlight's photon flux at the surface of the earth drops off very fast below 500 nm (see Figure 1.1). Thus, with natural sunlight as background, meta II is continuously photoconverted to rhodopsin, allowing the receptors of the frontal eye of *Ascalaphus* to maintain 90% of their pigment in the rhodopsin form (Hamdorf et al., 1973). In animals where the rhodopsin and metarhodopsin absorption spectra overlap to a greater extent, the percentage of visual pigment in the primary state declines. This would be the case for the squid, *Loligo peali,* whose pigment states are R493 and M500 and whose ratio of maximal extinction coefficients (metarhodopsin/rhodopsin) is 1.5 (Hubbard and St. George, 1958). Simple calculation shows that the photoequilibrium mixture of squid contains about 60% rhodopsin. This percentage remains relatively constant, irrespective of the spectral composition of the irradiating light, because the absorption spectra of the primary and meta states almost completely overlap. Similar considerations apply to *Limulus* ventral photoreceptors whose corresponding pigment states are R525 and M530 (Lisman and Sheline, 1976).

6.9 Early receptor potential

Now that the entire visual cycle has been treated in terms of its spectral intermediates, the second type of light-induced transitions will be discussed. These are the charge displacements, which parallel the sequence of spectral intermediates and which require electrophysiological techniques for their detection.

The early receptor potential (ERP) is a rapid potential change that can be recorded from photoreceptors only in response to a bright flash. The very intense flashes must be delivered within a short time interval, so that at least a few percent of the pigment is simultaneously photoactivated. The ERP can be recorded either intracellularly or, under appropriate conditions, extracellularly. Though the precise wave forms vary somewhat among species, the same underlying physical mechanism – molecular charge displacement – is reponsible for generating them.

The ERP is sometimes called a fast photovoltage. Because "fast photovoltage" is a nonspecific designation for all types of electrical effects (including ones that are thermal in origin), its use will be avoided in reference to photoreceptors.

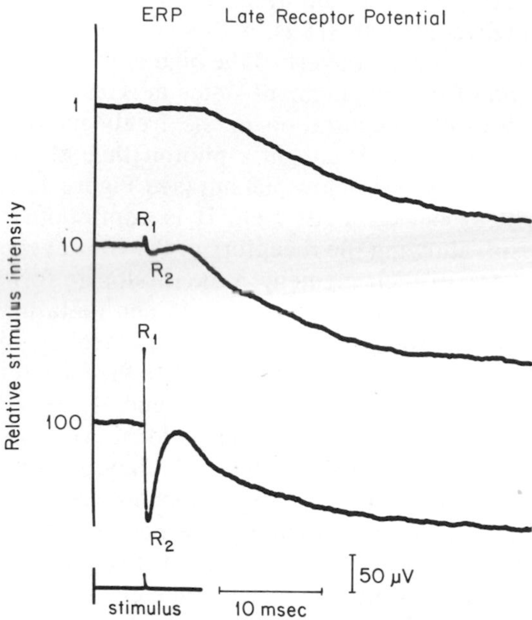

Figure 6.6. Extracellularly recorded early receptor potential, showing its characteristic wave form with its two phases designated as R_1 and R_2 and its temporal relationship to the late receptor potential (photoresponse). These records were obtained from the excised eye of the frog. Each trace represents the mass response from many photoreceptors and is caused by voltage gradients set up by extracellular currents. The currents responsible for the ERP are generated by the displacement of fixed charges on the membrane, and the currents of the photoresponse are due to a change in the ionic permeability of the membrane (see Chapter 7). An upward deflection in the recorded signal represents a corneally positive voltage gradient, corresponding to a current that flows from the inner segment layer to the outer segment layer in the subretinal space. For the top trace, the light intensity is sufficient to elicit a photoresponse but not an ERP. Note the 10-msec latency between the flash and the onset of the photoresponse. If the flash energy is increased by a factor of ten, as shown in the second trace, the ERP appears within the dead time. Further increases in flash energy lead to commensurate increases in the ERP. The amplitude of the photoresponse remains constant for all three traces because it saturates at much lower flash energies. The bottom trace was obtained with a flash that bleached about 10% of the pigment. The duration of the brief light stimulus is shown separately on the bottom left. (After Cone and Pak, 1971.)

6.9.1 Nature of the ERP response

Figure 6.6 illustrates the characteristic biphasic nature of the ERP, as recorded extracellularly in the frog. The initial corneal positive phase, designated R_1, is followed by a slower corneal negative phase, designated R_2. The action spectrum of both R_1 and R_2 closely match the absorption spectrum of rhodopsin (Cone, 1964; Pak and Cone, 1964). No measurable latent period exists between the stimulus and the rising phase of R_1. The amplitude of R_1 or R_2 linearly increases with flash energy, that is, with the number of photoactivated rhodopsin molecules, until the flash is so bright that photoequilibrium is achieved. Figure 6.6 illustrates this linear relationship over a limited intensity range. As reviewed by Cone and Pak (1971), the evidence is overwhelming that the ERP is produced by charge displacements within or very near to the oriented visual pigment molecule. In addition to the already cited properties, this conclusion is further supported by the ERP's insensitivity to fixatives and to ionic substitutions in the bathing solutions and, most importantly, by the ERP's correspondence with spectral transitions.

Because the ERP so closely reflects the state of the visual pigment, it is an alternate method for studying visual pigments under conditions where photometric methods are inappropriate. For example, the intracellularly recorded ERP has recently been used to study visual pigment kinetics and photoproducts in *Limulus,* the barnacle, and the turtle (Hillman et al., 1973; Fein and DeVoe, 1973; Minke et al., 1973; Lisman and Sheline, 1976; Hodgkin and O'Bryan, 1977).

6.9.2 Generating mechanism of the ERP

The mechanism whereby charge displacements within rhodopsin generate the ERP is illustrated in Figure 6.7. A schematic photoreceptor containing rhodopsin within its plasma membrane (as typical of vertebrate cones and invertebrate rhabdomeres) and within cytoplasmic vesicles (corresponding to the pinched off disks in rods) is shown. As with most proteins, rhodopsin is a charged molecule whose negative charges outnumber its positive ones at physiological pH. On the basis of its amino acid composition (Table 4.1), as many as about 50 negative and about 30 positive charges may exist on bovine rhodopsin. Their presence is indicated by the single positive and negative charge in the figure; their exact location and distribution being of little importance for the subsequent discussion. The fixed charges on the molecule contribute to the charge density carried on each membrane surface and are neutralized by diffusible counter ions in the surrounding aqueous

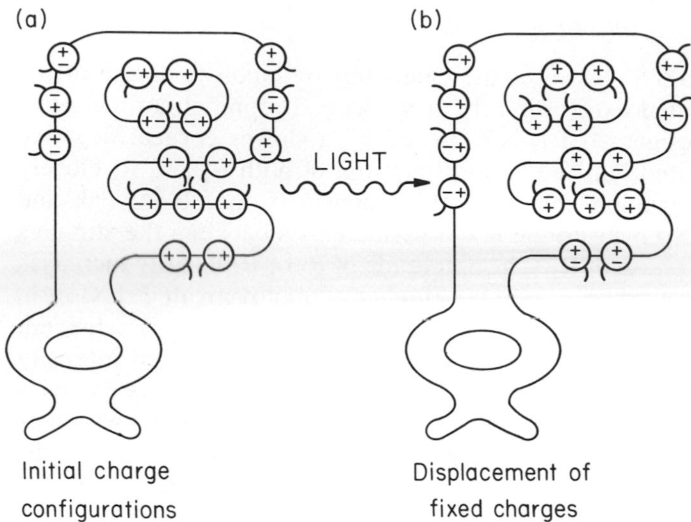
(a)
(b)
LIGHT
Initial charge configurations
Displacement of fixed charges

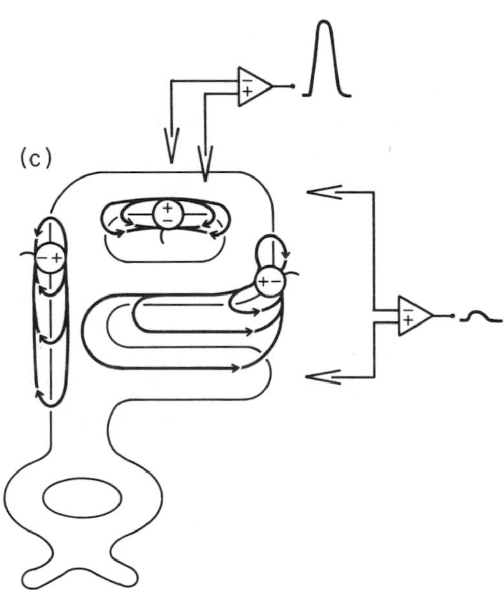
(c)
Induced current of mobile charges

solutions. The counter ions are mobile charges, which are set in motion by a voltage gradient, thereby creating a current. When, in response to a brief intense light flash, conformational changes within rhodopsins result in a simultaneous displacement of positive charges toward the cytoplasmic surface of the membrane, as happens for the onset of R_1, the charge densities of the cytoplasmic and external surfaces are slightly altered. The cytoplasmic side picks up a partial positive charge and the extracellular side becomes commensurately more negative. This causes an incremental voltage to appear across the region of membrane in which the rhodopsin is embedded. Note that *these charge displacements occur without any molecular reorientation and without any ionic current flow across the membrane*. The resulting incremental voltage, however, will initiate ionic current flow in the surrounding solutions. The diffusible anions and cations counterflow until the excess and debit charges are once again neutralized at the membrane–water interface. Positive current will flow from the incremental positive to the incremental negative side through the solutions and through the remainder of the membrane. Depending on the electrical properties of the membrane, the currents may flow appreciable distances in the extracellular medium. If this happens, the voltage drop created by them can be measured. Figure 6.7 illustrates the type of voltage signal one would record intracellularly and extracellularly for the given charge displacement. Because the specific resistance of ionic

Figure 6.7. Generation of an ERP signal by charge displacements. For a fuller explanation of this figure, consult the text. (*a*) Purely hypothetical representation of initial charge configurations on rhodopsin molecules when the receptor is in a dark-adapted state. The vectorial orientation of the molecules is indicated by a comma, which represents the sugar groups that face either the extracellular or the intradiskal solutions. (*b*) Simultaneous displacement of fixed charges by light so that positive charges move perpendicular to the plane of the membrane and toward the cytoplasmic interface. This charge displacement, which occurs without any change in the vectorial orientation of rhodopsin, alters the charge density of each membrane surface. (*c*) The incremental change in charge density sets into motion a flow of ions in the extracellular and cytoplasmic spaces. As the displaced fixed charges become neutralized by the diffusible ions, the currents diminish to zero. Simultaneous recordings of intracellular and extracellular potentials show a monophasic rise and decay (see wave forms). If the electrical properties of the plasma membrane are such that it does not resist current flow, then extracellular currents flow over only short distances, making extracellular recording of the ERP difficult. Large extracellular responses are possible when the membrane resistance is high and when all the photoactivated rhodopsins are located near one end of the cell.

solutions is much less than that of membranes, the extracellular voltage difference may be only about 100 μV, in contrast to the transmembrane potential of 1 to 10 mV. From the magnitude of the recorded ERP, it was concluded that the amplitudes of the R_1 and R_2 components are equivalent to the displacement of a single charge per visual pigment molecule moving over a distance of only a few angstroms (see the review by Cone and Pak, 1971). These are very small displacements indeed, and they may reflect the proton translocation spectroscopists observe on photoactivation (see Section 6.3). Using dielectric dispersion techniques, Petersen and Cone (1975) observed similar charge displacements with solubilized rhodopsin. In addition, Cafiso and Hubbell (1980) directly measured light-induced changes in the surface charge density of disk membranes, as required for the initiation of the aforementioned currents of mobile charges.

Currents induced by charge displacements exist in photoreceptors under all levels of illumination. However, at low intensities, they are undetectable. The simultaneous photoactivation of many molecules (and hence an intense light flash) is required to produce measurable effects. Rhodopsin molecules act in concert in generating the ERP because all of them share the same vectorial orientation with respect to the membrane. If rhodopsin molecules were randomly oriented in three-dimensional space, the generated currents would cancel each other, resulting in no detectable voltage. An additional requirement for ERP generation is that the charge displacement must have a component perpendicular to the plane of the membrane, otherwise it does not cause an incremental charge-density change on the membrane surface and, as a result, no current flows. This may be one of the reasons why some spectral transitions seem to be electrically silent. No detectable ERP signals could be attributed to the meta II → "retinal" and meta III → retinol + opsin transitions in rat (Cone and Cobbs, 1969) and for an uncharacterized reaction (possibly meta → rhodopsin) in *Limulus* ventral photoreceptor (Fein and Cone, 1973).

Note that currents due to charge displacement must complete their circuit across the very same membrane in which the displacement occurred. Currents initiated by pigment molecules within the isolated disks pass through the disk membrane with only negligible amounts, if any, passing through the plasma membrane. Thus, unless microelectrodes are inserted into the internal space of the disks, normal electrical recordings would not detect the ERP signal arising from rod disks. This was experimentally verified for receptors using intracellular (Murakami and Pak, 1970) and extracellular recording techniques (Rüppel and Hagins, 1973). It is also consistent with the observation that when the mass response of many cells is recorded (as in intact eyes or in isolated retinas), the ERP's action spectrum is nearer to that of the cone pigment. For example, in the frog, rhodopsin within rods contributes only a small fraction to the overall ERP response (Goldstein, 1968) even though it constitutes approximately 98% of the total visual pigment of the retina (Liebman and Entine, 1968).

One naturally wonders if the ERP plays any significant role in the process of visual excitation. Because the amplitude of the transmembrane-recorded ERP is undetectable with physiological stimuli (in turtle cones, the transmembrane voltage generated by a single photoactivated pigment is only about 10^{-4} μV for the ERP and about 30 μV for the late receptor potential; Hodgkin and O'Bryan, 1977), it can be stated with certainty that it is not the electrical signal that directly modulates information flow from the receptor to higher-order neurons. With intense flashes, however, charge displacements can create large enough signals to affect the receptor synapse (Hodgkin and O'Bryan, 1977).

6.10 Summary

It is the photolabile nature of visual pigments that makes them useful indicators of photon absorption. Their reliability is due to a molecular photoactivation step, which, acting as a trigger, initiates a sequence of dark reactions, initially confined to the pigment molecule and eventually including other cellular molecules and enzymes. The three types of light-induced transitions within rhodopsin include spectral shifts, charge displacements, and a transformation into a biochemically "active state." The latter represents rhodopsin's physiological function whereby the enzymatic reactions of phototransduction are begun. The transitions initiated by light absorption eventually have to be reversed to regenerate the initial pigment. The cycle of intermediates through which photoactivated rhodopsin progresses is called the visual cycle.

7 Photoreceptor excitation

By now the reader is well aware that the basic function of a photoreceptor is to transmit information to higher-order neurons about the intensity of light reaching an organism from its environment. *Individual receptors can be regarded as an engineer's "black box," which transforms light energy into an appropriate signal for successive nerve cells*. The ultimate function of a receptor could be fully described if its input–output relationships alone were given. Here input, of course, refers to the incident photons, which can be measured with great accuracy. The preceding chapters focused on the absorption of incident light by rhodopsin, with Chapter 6 describing the effects of photon absorption on rhodopsin itself. In this and subsequent chapters, we shall consider the receptor's output. Our goal is to try and understand the nature of the biochemical processes that intervene between photon absorption and the output signal. But, before delving into these aspects of physiology in Chapters 11 and 12, the reader needs to become familiar with the fundamental background material considered in Chapters 7–10.

7.1 Photoreceptor input–output relationship

One of the central concepts of neurobiology holds that neurons communicate with each other via synapses. The most commonly encountered synapses release chemicals, known as *synaptic transmitters*. It is by releasing these transmitters that one cell is able to communicate with its postsynaptic neighbors. Because photoreceptors are neurons with chemical synapses, their output is most likely also encoded in the release of their transmitters. In other words, for photoreceptors, the input–output relationship is simply a conversion of incident photons into transmitter release.

Direct measurement of synaptic transmitter release under physiological conditions is rather difficult and has not been accomplished with any photoreceptor to date. It would thus seem that a derivation of an input–output relationship is beyond our reach. However, another, nearly universal, neural property is of assistance: transmitter release is directly controlled by synaptic membrane potential. Therefore, by recording the variation of the membrane potential at the synapse, photoreceptor output could be indirectly surmised. Unfortunately, in most cases, it is technically difficult, if not impossible, to record intracellularly from the synaptic terminal. The vast majority of electrophysiological recordings have been carried out on other regions of the cell because these regions are larger and more accessible. So, in summary, the photoreceptor's output (unlike input) cannot be directly measured with our current technology. In most cases, the best that can be achieved is the measurement of changes in membrane potential at some site distant from the synaptic terminal.

7.2 Intracellular recording techniques

To record the electrical potential across a cell's plasma membrane, electrical contact must be made with the interior and the exterior. It is a simple matter to make an electrical contact with the cell's exterior, which is just its bathing salt solution. The problem is to achieve contact with the cell's interior without destroying the cell in the process. This is accomplished through the use of microelectrodes – glass capillaries that have been drawn to an ultrafine taper. The orifice at the tip of these microelectrodes is typically only a few tenths of a micron in diameter. The interior of the microelectrode is normally filled with a concentrated salt solution, such as potassium chloride (KCl), which, being an electrical conductor, provides a pathway for the electrical charges that move in response to a potential gradient. The glass walls of the electrode insulate the internal KCl solution from the solution that bathes the cell. Neurons are often damaged when impaled with a microelectrode, but sometimes they survive so that the electrical potential across the cell membrane can be measured for sufficiently long periods.

7.3 The photoresponse and the electrical properties of photoreceptors

Intracellular recordings have shown that photoreceptors, like other neurons, maintain their cytoplasm at a negative potential with respect to the outside of the cell. Depending on the particular photoreceptor, the resting potential varies between −30 and −70 mV. When we use the term *resting potential* in reference to a photoreceptor, we generally mean the membrane potential in the dark after the photoreceptor has had sufficient time to recover from any previous light stimulus.

7.3.1 *The response to light*

Electrical activity in many neurons is associated with action potentials, which occur on a time scale of milliseconds. In contrast, most photoreceptors do not produce action potentials. Whether or not they exhibit action potentials, all photoreceptors exhibit graded, slow changes in their membrane potential as a result of illumination. These potential changes occur on a time scale of tenths of a second to seconds and can be either depolarizing or hyperpolarizing (Figure 7.1). We shall refer to these slow light-induced changes in the membrane potential as *photoresponses* (also referred to as *generator* or *receptor potentials*). The photoresponse is the final expression of a series of biochemical reactions that were initiated by photoactivated rhodopsin. The entire process is generally called *photoexcitation,* or *phototransduction.* Confusion sometimes results from using the term "excitation" because the same word is invariably used to describe two distinct, albeit causally related, processes: one on the cellular and the other on the molecular level. Photopigment excitation in response to photon absorption is a molecular event. It initiates a sequence of reactions that eventually leads to photoreceptor excitation on the cellular level.

7.3.2 *Photon absorption by rhodopsin generates the light response*

That light absorption by rhodopsin is indeed responsible for the photoresponse can be tested directly in those photoreceptors in which both the absorption spectrum of the visual pigment and the spectral sensitivity of the photoresponse can be measured (see Chapter 5). If the spectral sensivity for the receptor potential closely matches the absorption spectrum of the visual pigment, it is reasonable to conclude that photoactivation of rhodopsin, and not other pigments, initiates the photoresponse. The overwhelming weight of evidence from these types of experiments unequivocally supports the conclusion that the absorption of light by visual pigment molecules initiates the events that lead to the receptor potential.

7.3.3 *Ionic permeability controls membrane potential*

What are these events that give rise to the light response? Before we can answer this question, the relevant concepts that have emerged from studies of other neurons need to be briefly reviewed.

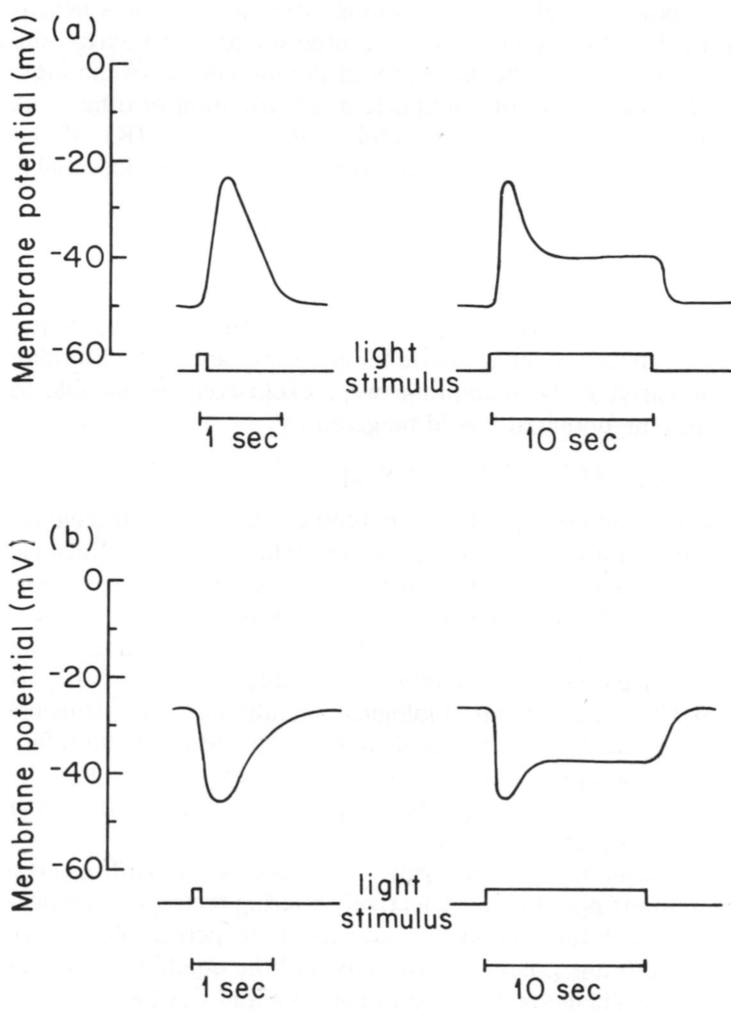

Figure 7.1. The two basic receptor potential types that have been observed with intracellular recording techniques: (*a*) depolarizing; (*b*) hyperpolarizing. As illustrated, most photoreceptors show a distinct difference in their response to stimuli of long and short duration. For short-duration stimuli, the response is typically a simple monophasic wave form. For long-duration stimuli, the response typically has an initial transient component that decays to a steady-state value. An upward deflection of the trace below each response indicates the duration of the light stimulus.

Generally speaking, the electrical potential difference across a neuronal membrane depends on the ionic concentration gradients across the membrane and the relative permeability of the membrane to the ions. We neglect the small, but not unimportant, contribution of other ions and focus our attention on sodium (Na) and potassium (K). If the membrane were exclusively permeable to K, its membrane potential E would be given by

$$E = E_K = (RT/F)\ \ln[(K)_o/(K)_i] \tag{7.1}$$

where E_K is the potassium equilibrium potential, $(K)_o$ the extracellular potassium activity, $(K)_i$ the intracellular potassium activity, R the universal gas constant, T the absolute temperature, and F the Faraday constant. Similarly, if the membrane were exclusively permeable to Na, the membrane potential would be given by

$$E = E_{Na} = (RT/F)\ \ln[(Na)_o/(Na)_i] \tag{7.2}$$

where E_{Na} is the sodium equilibrium potential, $(Na)_o$ the extracellular sodium activity, and $(Na)_i$ the intracellular sodium activity. Because $(Na)_o$ is greater than $(Na)_i$, E_{Na} is a positive number and corresponds to a transmembrane potential that is intracellularly positive with respect to the extracellular solution. On the other hand, E_K corresponds to an intracellularly negative transmembrane potential because $(K)_i$ is greater than $(K)_o$. In general, biological membranes and neuronal membranes in particular are permeable to both Na and K and therefore their membrane potential lies somewhere between E_{Na} and E_K, the proximity to either of these equilibrium potentials depending on the relative permeability to Na and K.

As a general principle, which is now well established, neurons control their membrane potential by selectively altering their ionic permeability. As the membrane becomes relatively more permeable toward one ion, the membrane potential moves toward the equilibrium potential for that ion. Whenever the membrane potential lies between E_{Na} and E_K, Na will tend to leak into and K will tend to leak out of the cell. Unless the cell compensates for the constant loss of K and gain of Na, the ionic concentration gradients will run down, E_{Na} and E_K will decrease toward zero, and the membrane potential will disappear. Neurons, including photoreceptors as well as other cells, have metabolically dependent enzymes, called *pumps,* that compensate for this passive leakage by pumping K into and Na out of the cell. It is generally agreed that the Na–K pump does not directly participate in the generation of electrical signals but rather has its effect by maintaining the ionic concentration gradients. This statement is not always true as we shall see shortly.

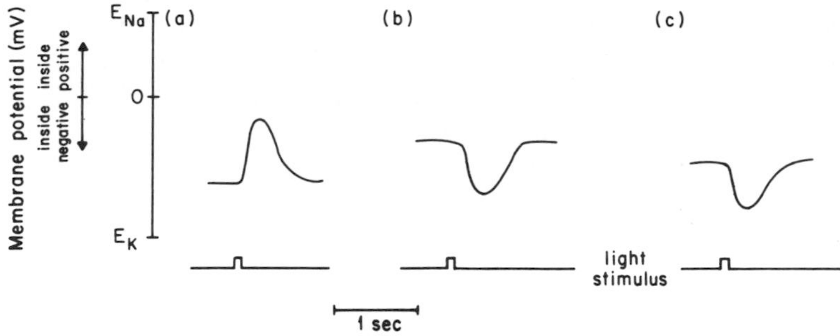

Figure 7.2. Idealized representation of the three basic types of permeability changes that have been found to underlie receptor potentials. (*a*) Increased Na permeability; (*b*) increased K permeability; (*c*) decreased Na permeability.

7.4 The basic photoresponse types

Now we shall return to the previous question about the identity of the events underlying the light response. Figure 7.2 shows three idealized models for their generation, representing situations that have been encountered in nature.

1. Figure 7.2*a* represents the situation for many invertebrate photoreceptors, especially those containing rhabdomeres. In the dark, these receptors are relatively more permeable to K than to Na, therefore their membrane potential is closer to E_K than E_{Na}. *A flash of light transiently increases Na permeability and thereby the cell transiently depolarizes toward* E_{Na}. The extent to which the cell transiently depolarizes will quantitatively depend on the relative Na-to-K permeability increase. It has been found that the magnitude of the permeability increase is graded with light intensity so that the photoresponse amplitude increases with light intensity (see Figure 8.5). The maximum amplitude of the light response will depend on the maximum value of the permeability ratio between Na and K. In no case can the membrane potential at the peak of the light response exceed E_{Na}. Fuortes and O'Bryan (1972) and Hagins (1972) provide reviews of the considerable experimental evidence that supports this description.

2. Two distinctively different mechanisms have been found to underlie hyperpolarizing photoresponses. The model illustrated in Figure 7.2*b* represents the mechanism that appears to generate hyperpolarizing photoresponses in the invertebrate photoreceptors of *Pecten* (Gorman and McReynolds, 1969, 1974; McReynolds and Gorman, 1970*a*, *b*). In the dark, the photoreceptor is permeable to Na and K and the

membrane potential lies between E_{Na} and E_K. As before, the exact value of the resting potential depends on the relative permeability to Na and K: *A flash of light transiently causes the cell membrane to become relatively more permeable to K than it was in the dark. The result is a hyperpolarization as the membrane potential moves toward* E_K. According to this model, the membrane cannot hyperpolarize beyond E_K.

3. Both vertebrate rods and cones hyperpolarize upon illumination (see Figure 7.2*c* and the review by Tomita, 1970). Unlike the photoreceptors previously described, the response of vertebrate photoreceptors is the result of a decrease in ionic permeability. In the dark, the receptor is permeable to both Na and K with the resting potential between E_{Na} and E_K. *The primary effect of light is to make the membrane less permeable to Na. The decreased Na permeability causes the membrane to hyperpolarize as the membrane potential moves closer to* E_K. See the articles by Hagins (1972) and Korenbrot and Cone (1972) for comprehensive reviews of the data supporting this description.

Figure 7.2 may appear to be incomplete because it does not cite an example of a depolarizing response that is primarily the result of a decrease in potassium permeability. At present there are no known examples of such a photoresponse.

7.5 Processes that further shape photoresponses

Actual intracellular records illustrating the three types of photoresponses just described are shown in Figure 7.3. A comparison of Figures 7.2 and 7.3 shows that the actual records closely resemble the idealized versions. However, closer inspection reveals that they are not exactly the same under all conditions or in all cells. For example, notice that in Figure 7.3 a very short duration transient appears with increasing light intensity. Its presence, as well as the presence of other variations among the receptors, is primarily due to two factors: (1) some receptors possess electrical properties that significantly modify their own photoresponse and (2) some photoreceptors directly or indirectly interact with their neighbors, thereby modifying each other's photoresponses. Neither of these two processes are considered to be part of phototransduction per se. At this point we shall enumerate some of the known mechanisms whereby receptors shape their own responses.

1. Not all the permeability changes in a photoresponse are a direct result of light. The plasma membranes of photoreceptors, as of most neurons, exhibit voltage-dependent changes in ionic permeability. For

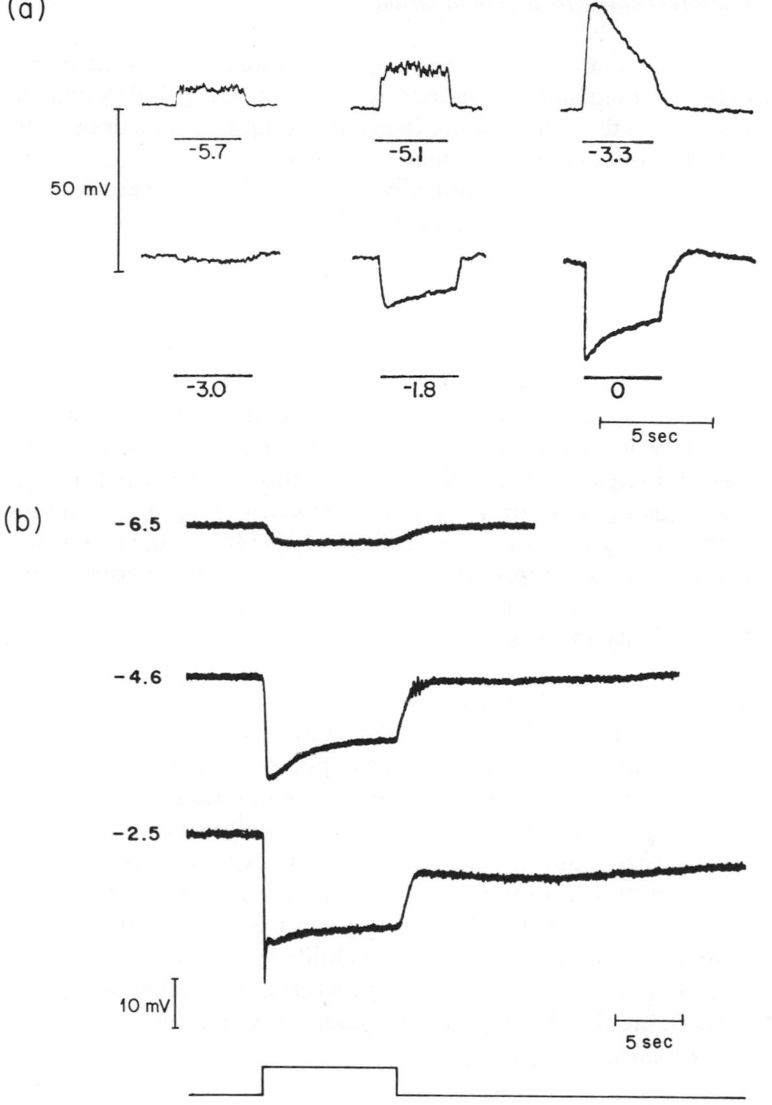

Figure 7.3. Examples of intracellularly recorded photoresponses. (*a*) Responses of a depolarizing cell (above) and a hyperpolarizing receptor (below) from the eye of the scallop, *Pecten irridians*, an invertebrate. The duration and relative intensity of the flash are shown below each response. (After McReynolds and Gorman, 1970*a*.) (*b*) Hyperpolarizing responses from a rod photoreceptor in the eye of the nocturnal lizard, *Gekko gekko,* a vertebrate. The duration of the stimulus is shown below the responses and the relative intensity of each stimulus is given to the left of each response. (After Kleinschmidt and Dowling, 1975.) For both parts, the relative intensity is given on a log scale.

example, in most neurons, including photoreceptors, membrane depolarization by itself can increase K-permeability. A permeability change by this mechanism does not require light (for examples, see Pepose and Lisman, 1978; Cornwall and Gorman, 1979).

2. The photoresponse may not always result from a permeability change toward a single ion. Protein molecules, which are the primary determinants of ionic permeability, are not perfectly selective for any one particular type of ion. Thus, a light-induced increase in sodium permeability is also accompanied by smaller increases in the permeability of other ions (Millecchia and Mauro, 1969; Brown et al., 1970; Brown and Mote, 1974). Furthermore, photoresponses in some cells, perhaps in all cells, result from more than one light-evoked permeability change. Detwiler (1976) has suggested that in *Hermissenda* photoreceptors light initiates processes that result in three distinct permeability changes, giving rise to a complex triphasic response, and in barnacle photoreceptors Hanani and Shaw (1977) have suggested that the photoresponse is composed of at least two distinct permeability increases; that is, a potassium permeability increase (P_K) in addition to the Na permeability increase (P_{Na}) previously described by Brown et al. (1970).

3. The metabolically driven pump, which pumps Na out of and K into the cell, can be electrogenic under some circumstances, where electrogenic means that on the average the pump can extrude net positive charge out of the cell, and thereby the membrane potential becomes more negative inside. Convincing evidence has been presented that in both barnacle and *Limulus* photoreceptors an electrogenic Na pump can contribute a prolonged hyperpolarizing component to the photoresponse (Koike et al., 1971; Brown and Lisman, 1972). In these photoreceptors, light increases Na permeability (see Figure 7.2), which results in an influx of Na. The resulting increase in intracellular Na is thought to activate the electrogenic Na pump, which in turn causes the cell to hyperpolarize transiently.

7.6 Summary

The photoreceptor's light response results from the absorption of light by the visual pigment molecules contained within the cell membrane. The overwhelming weight of experimental evidence indicates that the receptor potential is primarily the result of light-evoked changes in the ionic permeability of the plasma membrane. Whether the photoresponse is hyperpolarizing or depolarizing depends on two factors: (1) whether the permeability increases or decreases and (2) whether the primary ion involved is Na or K.

The preceding interpretation is modified by two factors. The first is that in those photoreceptors that have been studied in detail there are multiple light-evoked permeability changes and all these permeability changes contribute toward shaping the light response. Second, the permeability changes are not perfectly selective for one specific type of ion, but rather they allow several types to cross the membrane, each with different efficacy.

8 Adaptation

One striking aspect of the visual system is its ability to function over a very large dynamic range. For example, as shown in Table 1.2, the visual system of humans can function over a range of light intensities greater than a billionfold. Such a wide span is not unique to humans but occurs most likely for all organisms. The horseshoe crab is one of the few animals in which the range has also been measured – its dynamic range is nine log units (Barlow and Kaplan, 1971). The processes that enable the visual system to function over such a large range of light intensities are collectively referred to as *adaptation*.

We have all experienced our eyes' adaptive ability. When we leave a brightly lit street and enter a darkened theater, we are suddenly "blind" – we find our way among the rows by touch and feel. With time our vision improves so that what was previously invisible can eventually be seen. This increase in visual sensitivity with time is called *dark adaptation*. Should we leave the darkened theater after we have adapted to it and reenter the brightly lit street, our eyes must readjust to the excess light that initially blinds us. The loss of sensitivity to increased ambient light intensities is termed *light adaptation*.

Various mechanisms are used by the visual system to achieve such a huge dynamic range. These mechanisms occur at separate stages in the visual system. First, there are various mechanisms that, functioning together, serve to control the amount of light reaching the visual pigment molecules of our photoreceptors. Second, there are processes, within the photoreceptors themselves, that control the receptor's sensitivity. Finally, there are integrative processes, in the neurons proximal to the photoreceptors, that control visual sensitivity. Most of what follows will focus on the first two processes, with only very little said about the contribution of the integrative processes to adaptation.

8.1 Mechanisms that control the amount of light reaching the visual pigment

8.1.1 The pupil mechanism

We are all aware of our own pupil reflex, which controls the amount of light entering the eye. The human pupil area decreases by about a factor of 16 in going from darkness to bright light. Therefore, it can reduce the amount of light reaching the retina by 16-fold, or 1.2 log units. A greater decrease can be achieved in animals with slit pupils, such as cats. It is difficult to put an upper limit on the range of light control possible with a slit pupil because such a calculation depends on how well the edges of the slit can be opposed. Though only vertebrates and cephalopods are equipped with complex irises for pupil formation, simpler, but analogous, structures can also be found in many compound eyes.

8.1.2 Photomechanical movements – general considerations

Black-screening pigments (ommin and melanin granules) are ubiquitous in most eyes, where they primarily shield the photoreceptors from unwanted light. Not surprisingly, their ability to absorb light has been exploited in some organisms for controlling the amount of light reaching the visual pigment molecules. For this purpose, relative displacement must occur between the screening and visual pigments. Although it does not matter which of the two pigments is mobile, screening pigment migration is the more common event. Movement by the visual pigment involves movement by rhodopsin-containing membranes. These light-correlated migrations are, in general, called *photomechanical movements*.

8.1.3 Screening pigment movement

The location and direction of movement of screening pigments is quite variable among eyes. In vertebrate eyes, screening pigments are found solely in the cells of the pigment epithelium, where they can be either stationary or mobile. In contrast, within the cephalopod retina, mobile screening pigments are found mostly within photoreceptor cells. Figures 8.1*a* and *b*, respectively, show a tangential and radial view of a squid retina that had been light-adapted with a spot of light that illuminated a limited region of the retina. As can be seen, the normal location of the ommochrome granules in the unilluminated squid photoreceptors is at the base of the distal segment that contains the microvilli (see Figure 2.4). A sufficiently bright light causes the granules to migrate distally toward the tips of the receptors, where they absorb some of the incident light that might have otherwise traversed the rhabdom and been absorbed by the visual pigment. Their screening effect was found to be equivalent to placing a 0.6 log unit neutral density filter in front of the eye. In other words, the screening pigment caused a $10^{0.6}$, that is, a fourfold, reduction in the receptors' sensitiv-

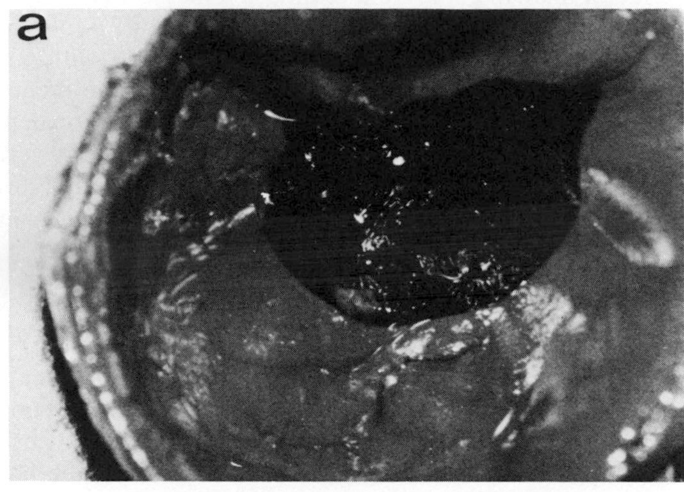

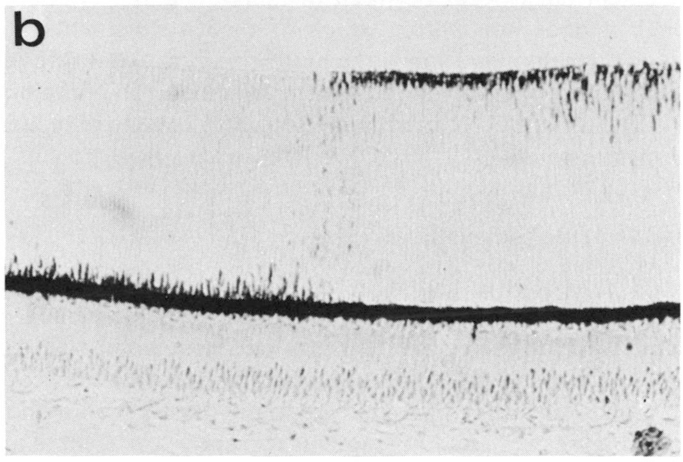

Figure 8.1. (*a*) Eyecup of a squid fixed after light adaptation to 25 μW/cm^2. Black spot corresponds to area illuminated. (*b*) Section of retina across the edge of the illuminated area. (After Daw and Pearlman, 1974).

ity. In a similar study, Hoglund (1966) investigated sensitivity changes associated with screening pigment movement in the eye of the moth, *Deilephila*. He did this by inserting through the pigment layer a fine glass fiber, which he used to test the sensitivity of the receptors independent of pigment position. Thus he was able to show that between 2

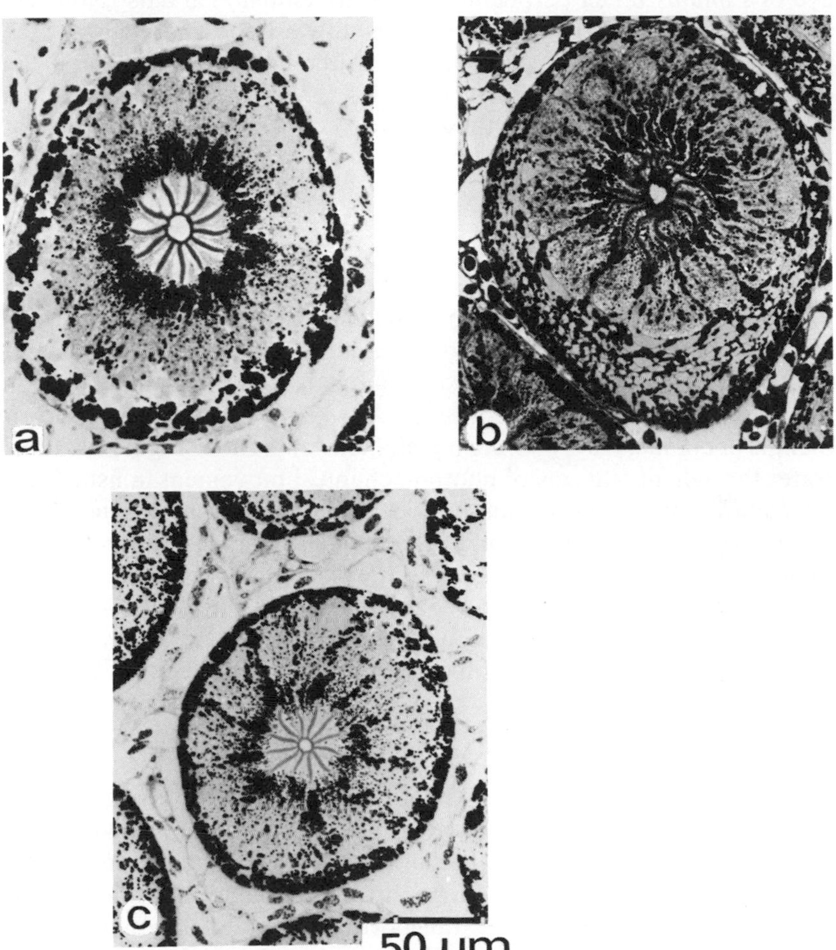

Figure 8.2 Radial pigment migration as a result of light adaptation in *Limulus* lateral eye. Light micrographs of ommatidia in three different states: (a) dark-adapted, (b) light-adapted for 15 min, and (c) light-adapted for 2 hr. Note that the pigment granules move into the rhabdom region only temporarily as a result of light adaptation. (After Barlow and Chamberlain, 1980.)

and 3 log units of sensitivity were controlled exclusively by screening pigment movement.

In vertebrate and cephalopod retinas, the direction of pigment migration is parallel to the photoreceptors' optical axis. In compound eyes, however, pigment migration occurs both parallel and perpendicular to the ommatidial axis. Figure 8.2 illustrates this with sections from the eye of *Limulus* taken perpendicular to the ommatidial axis. Note the radial movement of pigment granules toward the rhabdom, which occurred as a result of illumination. Although it has not yet been experimentally tested, pigment granules that approach the rhabdom during light adaptation are thought to reduce the intensity of light propagating through the rhabdom.

8.1.4 Receptor movement

In vertebrates, receptor movement is a reflection of axial extension or contraction of the myoid. All other subcellular structures remain essentially unaltered. Photoreceptor movements are prominent only in amphibians, fish, and birds; mammals lack them entirely. With the exception of a few genera (e.g., *Xenopus*), photoreceptor movement is accompanied by screening pigment migration. Figure 8.3 illustrates the salient features of photomechanical movement in fish. Light adaptation initiates elongation by rods and contraction by cones, with simultaneous vitreal migration of the melanin granules within the epithelial processes. On dark adaptation, all these are reversed. The net effect of light adaptation is to reduce the number of photons striking the rods and possibly also the cones. Unfortunately, the accompanying change in receptor sensitivity has not yet been reported.

8.1.5 Photomechanical movements – common features

Photomechanical movements are very slow processes, with long initial latencies. Their rates are on the same order of magnitude as axoplasmic transport in axons and other cells. For example, in squid, 5 to 15 min are required for the ommochromes to migrate over a distance of 300 μm, yielding an average transport rate of about 30 μm/min (Daw and Pearlman, 1974). The epithelial granules of vertebrates move an order of magnitude slower (Ali, 1975). The maximal rate for myoid contraction and extension is also about a few micrometers per minute (Ali, 1975; Burnside, 1976). Because of their slow rates and long latencies, photomechanical responses can mediate slow, not rapid, changes in sensitivity.

Photomechanical movements are initiated by photoactivated rhodopsin. At first this seems surprising because screening pigments themselves absorb light and it might be expected that their photon absorption would be the determining factor. The experimental evidence is clearly against that notion. Whether or not the mobile pigment is contained within the photoreceptors, the action spectrum for pigment migration is matched by the absorption spectrum of rhodopsin and not

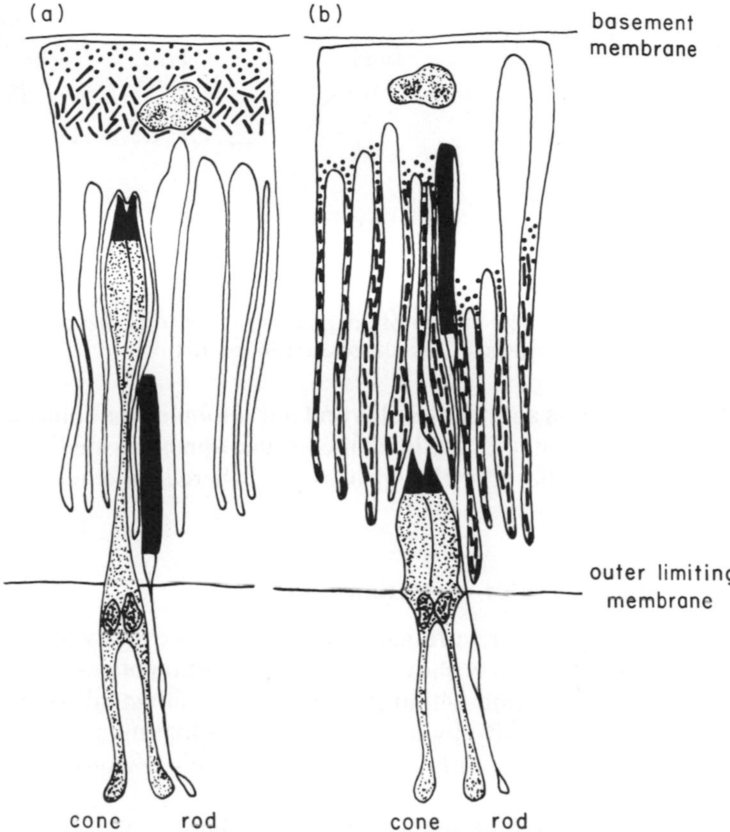

Figure 8.3. Schematic illustration of photomechanical movements in fish: (*a*) dark adaptation; (*b*) light adaptation. Fish retinal pigment epithelium cells possess long delicate apical projections that extend almost to the outer limiting membrane. In the fish (grey snapper), pigment moves into the projections in the light and reaggregates in the base of the cell in darkness. (After Burnside and Laties, 1979.)

by that of melanin or ommin. This was found to be the case in frogs (Liebman et al., 1969) and squid (Daw and Pearlman, 1974). Apparently light must first be absorbed by rhodopsin before any movement can occur. Virtually nothing is known about the processes that link light absorption with screening pigment movement.

The molecular mechanism of photomechanical movement is perhaps best understood for vertebrates (Burnside, 1976; the review by Burnside and Laties, 1979). Vertebrate photoreceptors are similar to other

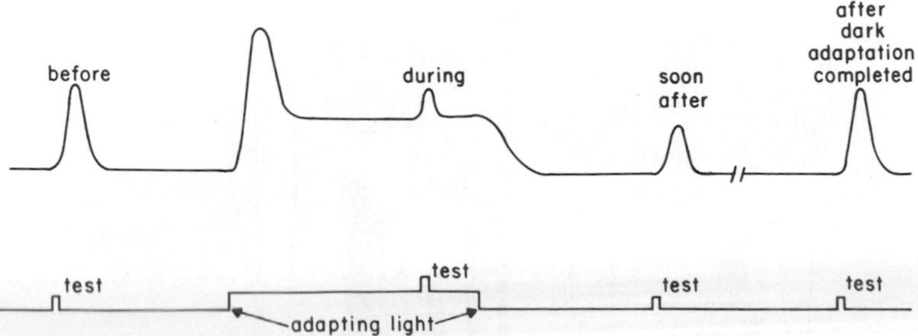

Figure 8.4. The effects of adaptation on the response to a constant-intensity test flash. See discussion in the text.

cells in relying on actin molecules and microtubules for contraction and extension of the myoid. Actin filaments also appear to mediate pigment migration into the epithelial processes, whereas the reverse movement is poorly understood.

8.2 Photoreceptor adaptation

Intracellular recordings from invertebrate and vertebrate photoreceptors have clearly shown that a large portion of adaptation is due to processes occurring within the receptors. Individual receptors can change their sensitivity by as much as 6 to 9 log units, a much wider span than that apparently achievable by the previously mentioned processes.

The manifestation of adaptation on the photoresponse is illustrated in Figure 8.4, which shows the effect of adaptation on the response to a constant-intensity test flash. Before the cell has been light adapted, the test flash elicits a certain response. The subsequent adapting light elicits a response that consists of an initial transient followed by a sustained steady state. During the steady state of the response to the adapting light, the test flash only elicits a small incremental response, indicating that the cell's sensitivity has decreased. Soon after the offset of the adapting light, the test response partially recovers, and with the passage of time, it fully recovers to its preadaptation value. These changes in photoreceptor sensitivity parallel the perceptual changes experienced in the aforementioned theater.

Changes in response amplitude to a constant-intensity test flash are of limited use in quantitative studies of adaptation. This is primarily because changes in amplitude can only be measured over about a 100-fold range (2 log units), whereas photoreceptor adaptation occurs over more than a millionfold (6 log units) range. In order to bridge this gap, changes in the photoreceptor intensity–response curve are often used to quantitate adaptation. Before describing how this is done, it will be worthwhile to digress at this point for a discussion of the intensity–response curve itself.

8.2.1 *Intensity–response curve*

The intensity–response curve is a plot of response amplitude versus stimulus intensity. In the preceding chapter, we described how both light-dependent and voltage-dependent permeability changes contribute toward shaping the light response. Thus, contributions from both of these permeability changes determine the shape of the intensity–response curve. The voltage-clamp technique allows one to record the photoreceptor light-response while keeping the membrane potential fixed, thereby allowing the current that results from the light-induced permeability change to be studied in isolation from the voltage-dependent currents. The intensity–response curve measured under voltage clamp, with the membrane potential fixed at the resting potential, only reflects the contribution of the light-induced permeability change.

Figure 8.5 presents the actual intensity–response curves of dark-adapted *Limulus* ventral photoreceptors and amphibian rods obtained under voltage clamp. The experimental protocol for obtaining the data is rather straightforward. The given receptor is impaled with electrodes and kept in darkness to reach a fully dark-adapted state. Increasingly brighter flashes are delivered and corresponding responses recorded. The time interval between successive test flashes must be long enough (with bright lights, the intervals may be minutes) to keep the state of dark adaptation unaltered throughout the experiment. The striking difference in the shape of the two curves is primarily a result of the difference in the coordinates along which each set of data is plotted. That this is so is shown by the fact that both sets of data are reasonably well fit by the solid curve which is a plot of the following equation:

$$a = a_{max}[I/(I + \sigma)] \tag{8.1}$$

where a is the light response amplitude, I the light intensity, σ the light intensity that results in a half-maximal light response, and a_{max} the maximal response amplitude. This *"rectangular hyperbolic"* relationship has been well known in biology for a long time and was first observed for retinal cells by Naka and Rushton in 1966. Both the Michaelis–Menten equation, used in enzyme kinetics, and the "Langmuir isotherm," used in binding studies, have the form of a rectangular hyperbola. It is common practice to plot intensity–

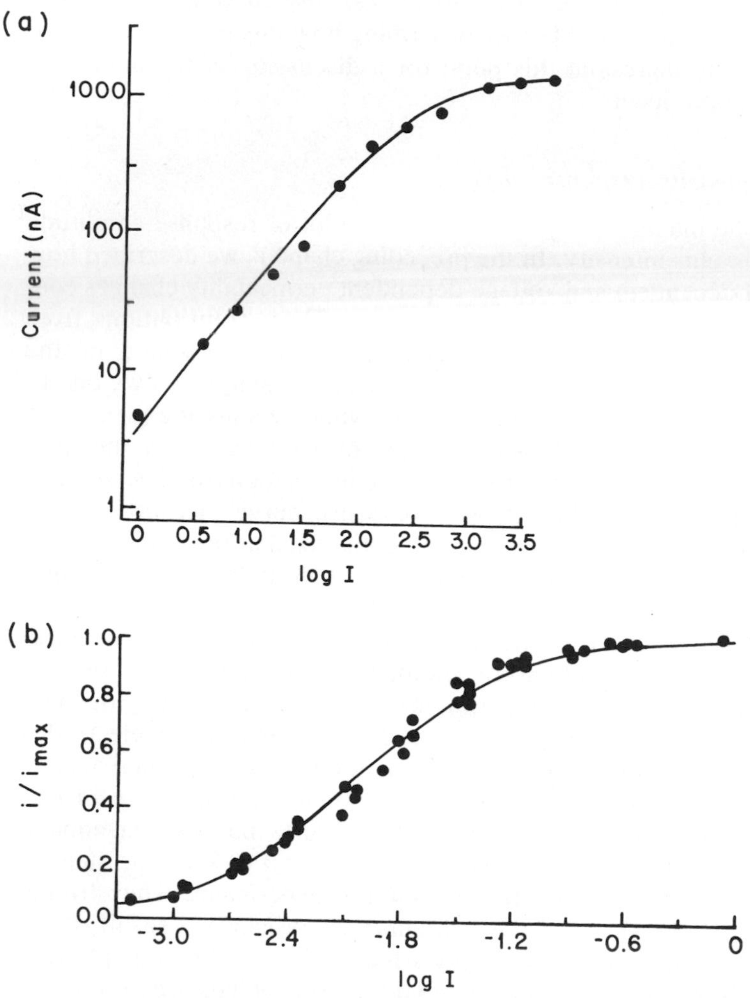

Figure 8.5. Voltage-clamp intensity–response relationship for: (*a*) *Limulus* ventral photoreceptor (after Lisman and Brown, 1975*a*); (*b*) vertebrate rod (after Bader et al., 1979.) Part (*a*) is a log–log plot of light-induced current versus relative intensity of test flash. (*b*) Normalized amplitudes of light-suppressed currents are plotted as a function of the log flash intensity. The continuous curves in (*a*) and (*b*) are plots of Equation (8.1).

response curves either on a semilogarithmic graph (Figure 8.5*b*) or on a log–log graph (Figure 8.5*a*). The log–log plot provides a clear visualization of the fact that the response amplitude is a linear function of light intensity only at the lower end of the response range.

In most cases, the light response is not usually measured under voltage clamp, but rather, the light-induced change in the *transmembrane potential* is measured as a function of light intensity. If the voltage responses were plotted on the ordinate in Fig. 8.5*a* or *b*, the fit between the data and Equation (8.1) would have been noticeably poorer. Most vertebrate and invertebrate photoreceptors exhibit an intensity–response curve that is reasonably well fit by Equation (8.1) or a modified version of it (Boynton and Whitten, 1970). It is not yet clear whether the voltage-dependent conductances can account for all the discrepancies between Equation (8.1) and the experimentally determined intensity–response curves of most photoreceptors.

Two features are noteworthy about the intensity–response curves of dark-adapted receptors. First, the response range is very limited. The response saturates only about 3 log units above the light intensity that elicits a barely detectable response. The critically important factor in determining the extent of the response range is the definition of a barely detectable response. Usually, in electrophysiological measurements, a threshold (criterion response amplitude) is defined and a response is considered detected when its amplitude exceeds this threshold. Typically, the criterion response amplitude is taken to be some multiple of the variance of the monitored variable (membrane current or voltage) in the absence of any stimulus. Because of the arbitrary nature of defining threshold, it sometimes becomes difficult to intercompare data from different laboratories.

Second, the light intensity that elicits the half-maximal response σ corresponds to a very low number of absorbed photons. It is only 30 to 50 absorbed photons in the rods of rats (Penn and Hagins, 1972), mudpuppies (Fain and Dowling, 1973), and toads (Fain, 1975). It is 10 to 100 times higher in cones (Baylor and Fuortes, 1970; Fain and Dowling, 1973). Because toad rods contain about 10^9 rhodopsin molecules, σ corresponds to a light intensity where only 1 out of every 10^8 rhodopsins is activated. In the ventral photoreceptor of *Limulus*, about 500 out of 10^9 rhodopsins need to be isomerized to obtain a half-maximal response (Brown and Coles, 1979).

8.2.2 Light adaptation and the intensity–response curve

The effects of light adaptation on the intensity–response curve are illustrated in Figures 8.6 and 8.7. The experimental data were obtained in a manner very similar to that shown in Figure 8.5. Following the adapting light's onset, the cell was allowed to achieve a steady state before its incremental responses to increasingly brighter flashes were recorded. As before, time intervals between test flashes were long

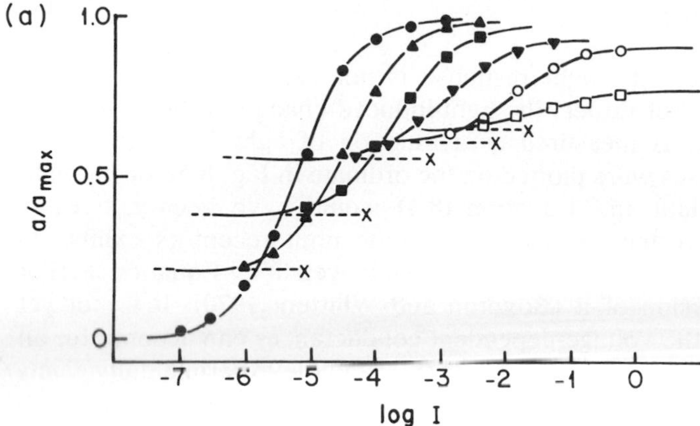

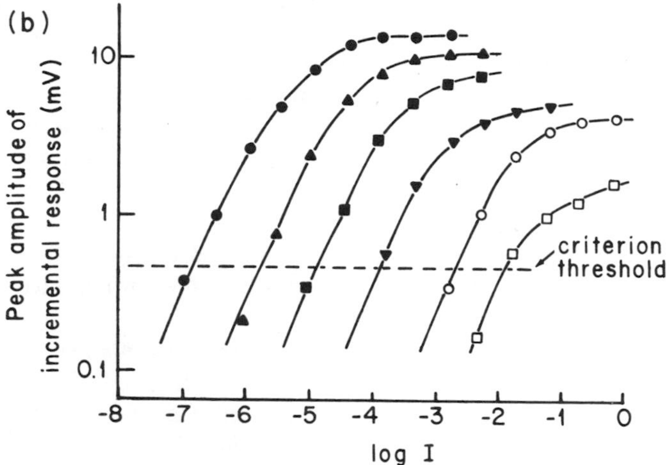

Figure 8.6. Voltage–intensity data from *Gekko* photoreceptors for responses to 0.1-sec test flashes in the dark-adapted state (●) and to 0.1-sec test flashes superimposed upon five different background intensities (I_B: $\log I_B = -5.1$, ▲; $\log I_B = -4.15$, ■; $\log I_B = -3.2$, ▼; $\log I_B = -2.2$, ○; $\log I_B = -1.7$, □. (*a*) On the ordinate are plotted peak amplitudes a of the responses measured from the dark-adapted resting potential and normalized with respect to the maximum peak amplitude a_{max}, obtained from the dark-adapted cell with a saturating flash. On the abscissa is plotted the intensity I of the test flashes. Dashed lines and crosses indicate the normalized plateau potentials prevailing for the various backgrounds. Solid lines are plots of Equation (8.2). (*b*) Replot of data from (*a*), but with the peak amplitude of responses in millivolts plotted on the ordinate. Peak amplitudes of incremental responses were measured from the prevailing steady level of membrane potential. The initial segment of all curves has a slope of 1. (After Kleinschmidt and Dowling, 1975).

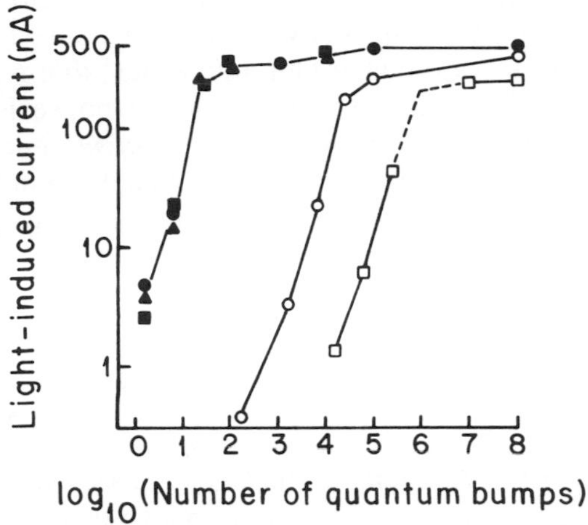

Figure 8.7. The effect of background illumination on the intensity–response function. The ordinate is the peak light-induced current and the abscissa is the stimulus energy relative to that necessary to evoke, on average, one quantum bump. The filled symbols (■, ●, ▲) are for separate intensity runs with the cell adapted to the dark. Between these runs, the cell was adapted to steady background illumination. Background illumination: ○, equivalent to $10^{5.05}$ quantum bumps sec^{-1}; □, equivalent to $10^{6.25}$ quantum bumps sec^{-1}. Data obtained from *Limulus* ventral photoreceptor voltage-clamped to its resting potential. (After Brown and Coles, 1979.)

enough not to change the state of adaptation. Figure 8.6*a* is a plot of absolute voltage versus light intensity. The response curves are both laterally and vertically shifted. The vertical shifts are caused by the fact that the incremental responses were superimposed on the steady-state response. Figure 8.6*b* replots the same data on a log–log graph, but now only the amplitude of the incremental response is plotted, the steady-state response being neglected. Similarly, Figure 8.7 shows the effects of light adaptation on the intensity–response curve measured under voltage clamp for a ventral photoreceptor of *Limulus*.

Figures 8.6 and 8.7 illustrate that, surprisingly, light adaptation does not dramatically change the shape of the intensity–response curve, and in fact, for most photoreceptors, a slightly modified form of Equation (8.1) fits the light-adapted intensity–response curve. Equation (8.1) is typically modified to Equation (8.2) by substituting the incremental response Δa for a in Equation (8.1):

$$\Delta a = \Delta a_{\max}[I/(I + \sigma)] \tag{8.2}$$

Examination of Figures 8.6*b* and 8.7 indicates that light adaptation has essentially only two effects on the intensity–response curve. (1) The curve is shifted to the right toward higher light intensities, that is, σ is increased. (2) The maximal obtainable incremental response is decreased. This decrease is commonly referred to as *response compression*. The major reason for the compression is that the background produces a steady-state response to which the incremental response must add. Equation (8.2) can be used to quantitate the relative contribution of response compression and increases in σ to adaptation. In the linear range of the intensity–response curve, I is much less than σ, and Equation (8.2) reduces to

$$\Delta a = (\Delta a_{max}/\sigma)I \qquad (8.3)$$

Examination of Figures 8.6*b* and 8.7 indicates that a_{max} decreases by at most a factor of 10, or 1 log unit, and σ increases by about a factor of 10,000 to 100,000, or 4 to 5 log units. In almost every photoreceptor studied to date, the decreases in sensitivity resulting from increases in σ are quantitatively greater than those resulting from decreases in a_{max} (response compression).

8.2.3 *Kinetics of light and dark adaptation*

With dark adaptation sensitivity rises and with light adaptation it falls. Therefore, the two processes might be thought of as the reverse of each other. Indeed, intensity–response curves and thresholds on dark adaptation shift in a manner analogous to light adaptation but in a reverse direction.

The two processes are not, however, the same reel of events, run either forwards or backwards. First, careful quantitative analysis indicates that conditions cannot be manipulated so that both adaptations precisely mimic each other (Fein and DeVoe, 1973; Kleinschmidt and Dowling, 1975). Second, the kinetics of light and dark adaptation are quite different. As a general truism, for any given receptor, light adaptation is much faster than dark adaptation. This second point is illustrated in Figures 8.8 and 8.9 for the ventral photoreceptor of *Limulus*. It can be seen in Figure 8.8 that the primary decrease in sensitivity associated with light adaptation occurs on a time scale of seconds, whereas in Figure 8.9 dark adaptation takes on the order of minutes. Part of the difference in the time course between the two figures results from the difference in the light intensities used in each experiment. This points out a basic problem in trying to specify the time course of light and dark adaptation; the kinetics of both processes are highly dependent on stimulus intensity. One feature of Figure 8.9

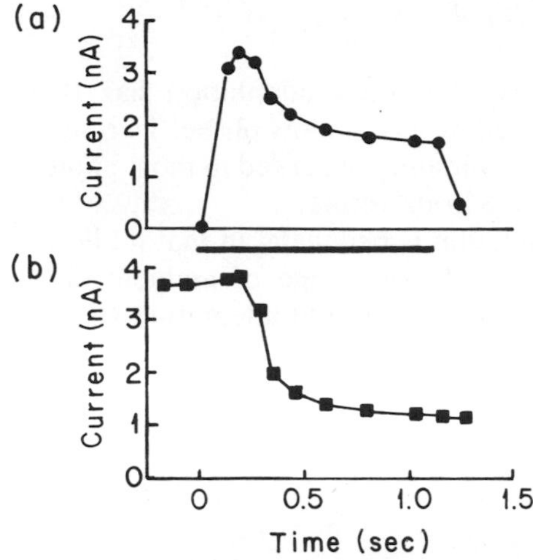

Figure 8.8. Changes in amplitude of responses to test flashes during an adapting stimulus, as recorded in the ventral photoreceptor of *Limulus*. (*a*) The response to the adapting stimulus. (*b*) Amplitude of the response to a brief test flash given at different times, where the bar represents the duration of the adapting stimulus. Zero time marks the onset of the adapting stimulus. (After Lisman and Brown, 1975*a*.)

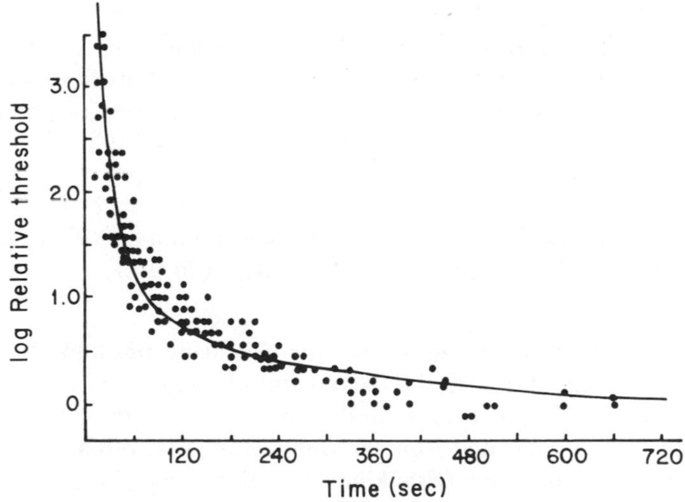

Figure 8.9. Log relative thresholds of the *Limulus* ventral photoreceptor light response after single intense flashes delivered at time zero. Dark adaptation occurs in two phases, an initial rapid phase and a later slow phase. The smooth curve was fitted by eye to give a rough estimate of the time constants, which are 20 sec for the fast phase and 270 sec for the slow phase. (After Fein and DeVoe, 1973.)

deserves further comment; that is, that dark adaptation has two phases, an initial rapid phase, followed by a later slow phase. Two such components of dark adaptation are commonly observed in most photoreceptors, including those of the vertebrate retina.

It is quite obvious that light adaptation is beneficial in that it allows the visual system to function over a broad range of ambient light intensities. And intuitively it would seem that light adaptation should be a relatively rapid process in order to facilitate rapid adjustments to increases in ambient illumination. The reason for the slow rate of dark adaptation is puzzling because it is not at all obvious how it could be beneficial to an animal.

8.2.4 The role of visual pigment in adaptation

Just as with excitation, one can ask whether light adaptation results from the absorption of light by rhodopsin. It might be that adaptation is initiated when light is absorbed by a photoproduct rather than by rhodopsin itself. In those instances where this possibility has been tested, it has turned out that the action spectra of both excitation and adaptation matches the absorption spectrum of rhodopsin (for example, see Lisman and Strong, 1979).

At this point it is appropriate to ask the question, how does the absorption of light by rhodopsin bring about adaptation? In all photoreceptors, photon absorption converts rhodopsin to a series of photoproducts which then decay as rhodopsin is regenerated (Chapter 6). Perhaps adaptation is linked to the concentration of a specific photoproduct (rather than to light absorption by that photoproduct) or to the concentration of those rhodopsin molecules that did not absorb a photon. Each of these alternatives shall be considered in turn.

Is there a linkage between sensitivity and a specific photoproduct? There have been suggestions that a component of adaptation in retinal rods is associated with one or more of the photoproducts of rhodopsin (for example, see Donner and Reuter, 1968). However, other studies have not supported this view (Frank and Dowling, 1968; Frank 1969, 1971). Recently, Brin and Ripps (1977) developed a procedure that may completely settle this question. They used hydroxylamine to accelerate greatly the photochemical reactions in the isolated skate retina. They found that whereas the photochemical reactions were greatly accelerated by hydroxylamine, there was no significant effect on the rate of recovery of rod sensitivity. Their techniques might be profitably applied to any retina where photoproducts are suspected of being involved in adaptation. Adaptation in those invertebrate photoreceptors that have been studied also appears to be independent of the photoproducts of rhodopsin (for example, see Seldin et al., 1972; Fein and DeVoe, 1973).

Is there a linkage between sensitivity and rhodopsin concentration? According to a simple interpretation of this alternative, threshold should rise whenever the number of rhodopsin molecules decreases in the cell. This is because with fewer molecules, fewer photons are caught. In other words, the cells' *quantum catch* is lowered. As a result, threshold is inversely proportional to the fraction of unbleached rhodopsin molecules. For example, a 50% decrease in concentration would result in a twofold elevation of threshold. In as much as decreases in rhodopsin concentration greater than 90% are uncommon at physiological intensities, this mechanism cannot be considered to make more than a tenfold (1 log unit) contribution to adaptation. Because adaptation changes sensitivity by much more than one log unit in most photoreceptors (see Figures 8.6 and 8.7), a change in quantum catch can contribute only a *small component* to the overall process of adaptation. Such a small contribution in fact has been experimentally verified in a number of invertebrate photoreceptors (see review by Hamdorf, 1979).

The situation for vertebrate rods is more complicated than for the invertebrate receptor. It turns out that, under certain circumstances, large changes in sensitivity can be linked to the amount of bleached rhodopsin. Dowling (1960) and Rushton (1961) showed that there was a linear relationship between the amount of bleached rhodopsin and the logarithm of the threshold *during the slow component of dark adaptation*. The experiments of Dowling, on the rat, and Rushton, on humans, could not establish whether the desensitizing effect occurred in the photoreceptor. This was because their measure of threshold (electroretinogram-b wave in the rat, subjective threshold in humans) involved higher-order neurons. More recently (see Figure 8.10), it has been shown that a logarithmic relationship exists between receptor sensitivity and bleached pigment for several vertebrate species. It is not clear in these experiments whether the desensitization results from an increase in the amount of bleached pigment (that is, opsin) or a decrease in the amount of unbleached pigment. Numerous suggestions have been made to explain why the bleaching of small amounts of rhodopsin should produce such large changes in sensitivity in vertebrate rods (see discussion in Gouras, 1972). However, these suggestions have not as yet led to any definitive experiments to test their validity.

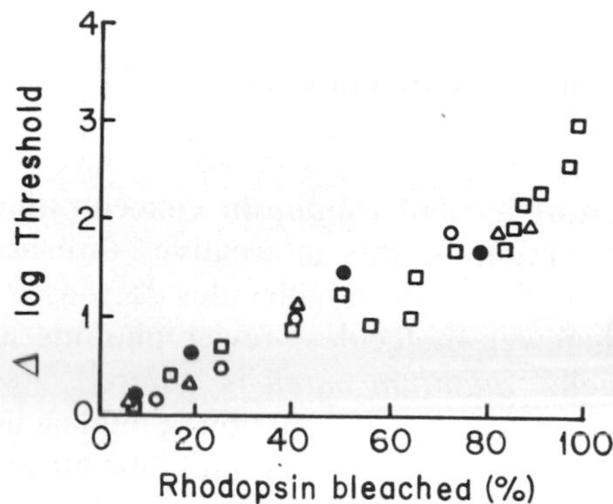

Figure 8.10. Relationship between the concentration of bleached rhodopsin and the threshold of receptor responses of isolated retinas of axolotl (●), frog (○, △), and rat (□). Recall that in isolated retinas pigment regeneration does not occur. (After Grabowski and Pak, 1975.)

8.3 Integrative processes and adaptation

There are numerous examples whereby higher-order neurons contribute to adaptation. One particular case is of special interest because it occurs in humans and entails integration of information from different types of receptors, rods and cones. When the time course of dark adaptation is followed, after an adapting light that bleaches significant amounts of visual pigment in both rods and cones, the results shown in Figure 8.11 are obtained. Indirect experimental evidence indicates that the observed kinetics are largely, if not solely, attributable to the receptors themselves. Following dim-adapting lights that photoactivate only rods, visual threshold recovers in two stages: a fast initial stage, which, in this figure, takes less than 1 min, followed by a slower phase that takes about 20 min (see discussion in Section 8.2.4). As the adapting illumination is increased, cones are increasingly stimulated and begin to contribute to dark adaptation. Their recovery is much faster than the rods', and as a result, a prominent plateau is observed in the recovery curves. At this plateau, visual threshold is solely determined by the cones. The rods do not contribute because their thresholds exceed those of cones. With the brightest adapting light employed in Figure 8.11, more than 15 min elapses before the rods begin to mediate vision, and more than 30 min is required for them to regain their absolute threshold. In contrast, the cones completely recover within 5 to 10 min. This is only one manifestation of how the

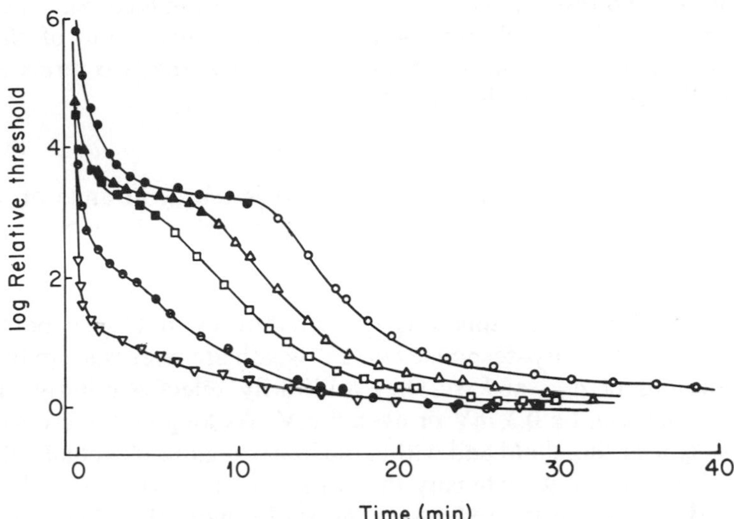

Figure 8.11. The course of human dark adaptation following different degrees of light adaptation. Threshold was the intensity of the violet test light that enabled an opaque black cross to be seen. The log relative adapting intensities were: ●, ○, 3.18; ▲, △, 2.17; ■, □, 1.87; ⊖, 1.16; ▽, 0.00. The intensities used were sufficient to bleach from 0.35 to 99.6% of the rhodopsin. The filled symbols indicate that a violet color was apparent at threshold, whereas the open symbols indicate that it was colorless. (After H. B. Barlow, 1972.)

human visual system extends its dynamic range by using the rods and cones to mediate vision at different light intensities.

8.4 What constitutes adaptation?

It may seem strange to raise the question of what constitutes adaptation at the end of a chapter on adaptation, but our reason for doing so was simply to avoid the trap of a restrictive definition, which would limit the processes being discussed. If we define the sensitivity of the photoreceptor as the response amplitude in volts per absorbed photon, anything that alters this sensitivity can be thought of as adaptation. However, by this definition, any process that limits the amount of light reaching the photoreceptor would not constitute adaptation. In order to include the latter processes, one must think in terms of the sensitivity of the eye and not of photoreceptors.

Sensitivity and threshold are common terms and, indeed, have been used regularly throughout this book. A precise discussion of their relationship is therefore in order. Mathematically, the two terms are reciprocally related to each other, that is,

$$\text{threshold} = 1/\text{sensitivity} \tag{8.4}$$

Thus, in terms of Equation (8.1), threshold is σ/a_{max} in units of absorbed photons per millivolt or, if the light intensities have not been calibrated for absorption, in units of incident photons per millivolt. Operationally, however, electrophysiologists and psychophysicists do not determine threshold this way – often they do not even bother generating the intensity–response curves, which are necessary in finding the values of a_{max} and σ. They arbitrarily select a criterion response, which can be 0.5 mV or even 5 mV. As long as the criterion response is near threshold and within the linear region, its actual value is immaterial. The light intensity that corresponds to this criterion is then an expression of the receptor's threshold. Note that, because of the linear relationship at the bottom of the dynamic range, the mathematical and operational procedures for determining threshold are equivalent. The essence of the operational procedure can be illustrated by a simple graphical analysis. Using the data of Figure 8.6*b,* we can draw a horizontal line at a chosen response amplitude so that the line intersects all the intensity–response curves. The stimulus intensity corresponding to each intersection then gives the relative threshold. To convert these relative thresholds to absolute thresholds the calibration of the light source must be known.

It is also possible to make an even more restrictive definition of photoreceptor sensitivity. One can define the sensitivity in terms of the position of the intensity–response curve along a scale of light intensity. What is typically done is to use σ [the light intensity that gives a half-maximal light response; see Equation (8.1)] as a measure of the sensitivity. According to this definition a change in the amplitude of the light response could occur without a change in sensitivity. How this might occur can be seen with reference to Equation (8.1). If a_{max} changes, the response amplitude changes without a change in σ, the sensitivity. All these definitions are commonly used in the scientific literature.

8.5 Summary

Photoreceptor sensitivity is ultimately related to visual pigment concentration because it determines the probability that an incident photon is absorbed. In the retinal rods of vertebrates, the bleaching of rhodopsin produces change in sensitivity much larger than can be explained by changes in quantum catch. The mechanism responsible for this effect is unknown. For all photoreceptors (vertebrate and invertebrate), there are large components of adaptation that are *not* correlated with any photometrically measurable changes in the visual pigment. However, it should be kept in mind that there may be changes in the visual pigment molecules that are not reflected in a change in the absorption spectrum, and such changes might be correlated with adaptation.

9 Response to single photons

Now that we have described the photoresponse and the effect of adaptation on it in the last two chapters, our aim is to understand the entire process in molecular terms. To accomplish this, we must first examine the additional properties of the photoresponse that reveal the nature of these underlying processes. This and the following chapter will be devoted to these properties. Specifically, in this chapter we shall deal with the attempts to relate the photoresponse to the quantum nature of light.

As the reader might guess, the quantum nature of light is most directly evident at low light intensities, where a light stimulus consists of a small number of photons. Furthermore, we know that there is a lower limit to the threshold of vision because a photoreceptor can do no better than respond to a single photon. Therefore, measurements near the absolute visual threshold would be expected to yield information about how the photoisomerization of an individual rhodopsin molecule is transformed into the light response.

9.1 Psychophysical determination of absolute visual threshold

Hecht and co-workers (1942) measured the absolute visual threshold in humans. They estimated the number of photons absorbed by the photoreceptors at absolute threshold and thereby concluded that a threshold flash was seen when a quantum of light was absorbed by each of 5 to 14 rods. Their findings clearly indicated that a human rod responds with a detectable signal to a single photon. What is the actual photoresponse under such conditions? The answer had to wait many decades before electrophysiological techniques made it possible to record from individual receptors.

9.2 Photoresponses near absolute threshold

By recording intracellularly from the dark-adapted lateral eye of *Limulus,* Yeandle (1958) observed fluctuations in membrane potential that resulted from randomly occurring waves of depolarization, which were irregular in size and are commonly referred to as *discrete waves*. Even if care were taken to eliminate all sources of light, discrete waves would still be present, indicating that these fluctuations were spontaneous events. Yeandle also discovered that illumination of the photoreceptor led to the production of similar discrete waves. At low light intensities, the average frequency of light-induced discrete waves increased linearly with light intensity (Fuortes and Yeandle, 1964; Adolph, 1964). Figure 9.1 shows an example of *spontaneous* and *light-evoked discrete waves* and their dependence on light intensity. If a *Limulus* photoreceptor is stimulated by a dim flash, the number of waves evoked varies randomly with time, obeying approximately a Poisson distribution (Yeandle, 1958; Fuortes and Yeandle, 1964; Adolph, 1964). Because at low light intensities the number of photons that a flash delivers is not constant but randomly fluctuates about a mean following Poisson statistics, it was suggested that the variability in discrete-wave occurrence resulted from the inherent variability in photon absorption. The actual statistics of their occurrence suggested that light-induced discrete waves were single-photon events (Yeandle, 1958; Fuortes and Yeandle, 1964). If they are truly single photon events, then one wave should result when the receptor absorbs about one photon. Borsellino and Fuortes (1968) extended the statistical analysis by estimating the average number of photons absorbed with each stimulus. With some uncertainty, they concluded that the light-evoked discrete waves are indeed the result of the absorption of about one quantum of light.

Light-induced discrete waves have been recorded from photoreceptors of the locust (Scholes, 1965), fly (Kirschfeld, 1965), leech (Walther, 1965), spider (DeVoe, 1972), *Limulus* ventral eye (Millecchia and Mauro, 1969), *Drosophila* (Wu and Pak, 1975), and toad (Yau et al., 1977). The underlying conductance change producing these waves varies from about 50,000 picoSiemens (pS) in *Limulus* to 30 pS in toad. Based on this limited survey of the animal kingdom, it appears that discrete waves are fundamental to the process of phototransduction. In some receptors, discrete waves have not yet been experimentally recorded, most likely because the magnitude of the events is below the sensitivity of the measuring technique. As will be discussed in the next section, the quantitative measurements in the locust (Lillywhite, 1977) and toad (Baylor et al., 1979*a*) reconfirm that light-induced waves are indeed single-photon events. Because of the association between wave production and photon absorption, light-induced discrete waves have often been referred to as *quantum bumps*, or, simply, *bumps*.

(a)

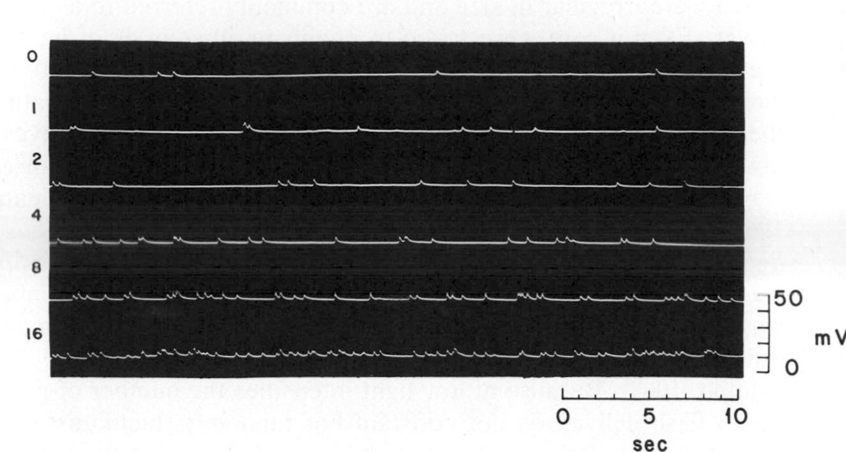

(b)

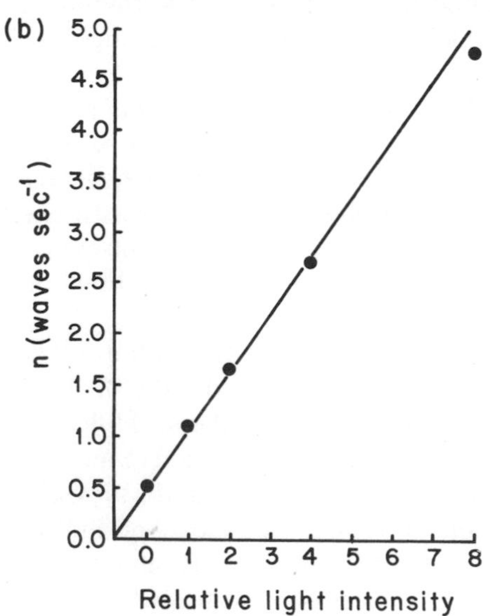

Figure 9.1. Spontaneous and light-evoked discrete waves recorded from *Limulus* lateral eye. (*a*) Intracellular recordings of discrete waves during constant illumination at the relative light intensities given by the number at the left of each record. The record designated as 0 was obtained in the dark and hence represents spontaneous activity. (*b*) Dependence of discrete-wave frequency on relative light intensity. The data fall approximately on a straight line. (After Fuortes and Yeandle, 1964.)

9.3 Quantum efficiency of bump production

To determine how reliable a detector a photoreceptor is, the *quantum efficiency of bump production* can be measured. The quantum efficiency of bump production is simply the probability that an absorbed photon will produce a discrete event. Lillywhite (1977) found that the quantum efficiency of bump production was greater than 0.59 for the retinular cells of the locust, and Baylor et al. (1979*a*) obtained a value of 0.5 in toad rods. Remembering that the quantum efficiency for photoactivating rhodopsin is about 0.7 (Section 4.7), these findings suggest that the photoisomerization of a chromophore will produce a quantum bump with nearly 100% probability.

9.4 The nature of spontaneous discrete waves

Spontaneous discrete waves appear to be similar to the light-induced waves except that light is not required for their occurrence. It may have occurred to the reader that because photoactivation of the visual pigment molecule triggers a discrete wave, it may be that the spontaneously occurring discrete waves are triggered by *thermal isomerization of rhodopsin*. Such a prediction would generate credence if both the rate and temperature dependence of the two processes could be shown to be identical. Unfortunately, both the rate and temperature dependence of the thermal isomerization of rhodopsin are nearly impossible to measure because rhodopsin is so stable (see Section 4.4). Therefore, experimenters are forced to test this prediction solely on the basis of the temperature dependence of discrete wave occurrence. Baylor and co-workers (1980), whose work is the most recent example of this line of research (Adolph, 1968; Srebro and Behbehani, 1972) found that the temperature dependence in toad rods corresponds to an activation energy of 22 kcal $mole^{-1}$ for the production of discrete waves. How does this value compare with the activation energy for thermal isomerization? If we assume that thermal isomerization proceeds by the same pathway as photoisomerization, then the activation energy of thermal isomerization is 45 kcal $mole^{-1}$, the activation energy for bathorhodopsin formation (see Section 6.3). Clearly, the temperature dependence of spontaneous wave production and thermal isomerization are nonidentical, suggesting no causal relationship between them. This conclusion has been further reinforced by the recent observation that chemicals, which are unlikely to act directly on rhodopsin, profoundly increase the rate of spontaneous discrete waves (Fein and Corson, 1979, 1981).

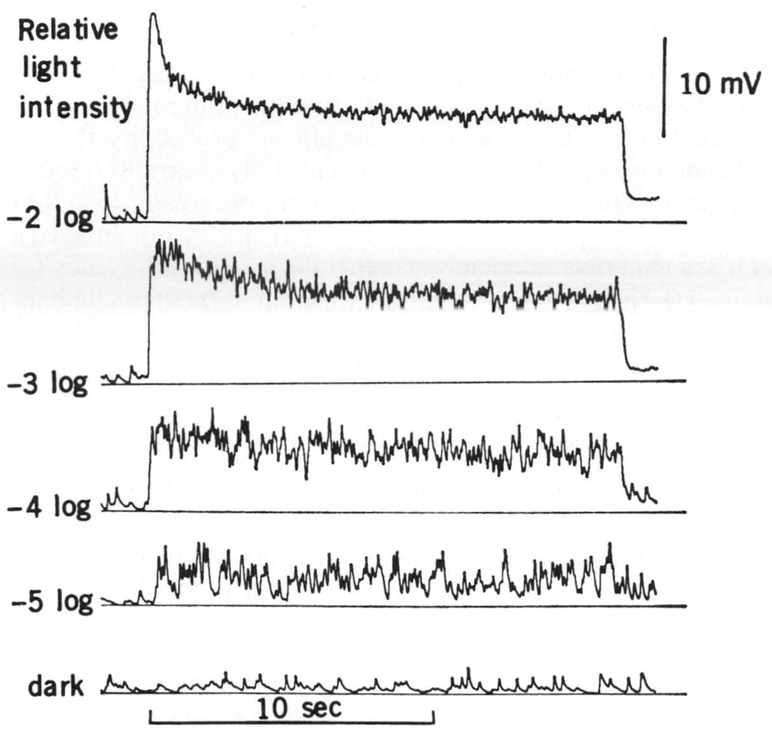

Figure 9.2. Representative recordings of light response at different light intensities. Intracellular recordings were from *Limulus* lateral eye. (After Dodge et al., 1968.)

If isomerization of rhodopsin is not the source of spontaneous discrete waves, then what is? No one yet knows, but fluctuations in the basal activity of the enzymes anywhere along the early stages of the phototransduction pathway could easily explain the occurrence of spontaneous discrete waves.

9.5 Does the light response result from a summation of quantum bumps?

With the discovery of quantum bumps, it became apparent that the receptor potential discussed in Chapters 7 and 8 might result from the *summation of bumps*. This notion was first carefully tested in *Limulus* lateral photoreceptors by Dodge et al. (1968). Figure 9.2 shows the type of data they analyzed to test this idea. At each light intensity, during the steady-state component of the response, the receptor potential fluctuated around some mean amplitude. They assumed that the receptor potential resulted from the summation of individual bumps, and from measurements of the mean and variance of the receptor potential during the steady state, they could calculate the rate of occurrence and the mean amplitude of these bumps. They found that initially the bump rate increased linearly with light intensity, but with increasing intensity, the rate departed from strict proportionality, indicating a reduced quantum efficiency of bump production. The steady-state bump size decreased continuously with light intensity. The decrease in bump size was found to be responsible for the eventual decrease in response variance with increasing mean amplitude of the receptor potential seen in Figure 9.2. They arrived at two principal conclusions from their study: first, that the assumption was correct, the receptor potential does indeed arise from the summation of discrete bumps; and second, that the average size of a bump decreases markedly as the ambient light intensity is increased, and this is the primary mechanism of light adaptation (see Chapter 8). This type of analysis was applied to *Limulus* ventral photoreceptors (Wong, 1978) and *Drosophila* photoreceptors (Wu and Pak, 1978), confirming and extending these ideas. Preliminary experiments with toad rods also suggest that the steady light response results from a summation of bumps (Baylor et al., 1979*a*). Additional experiments are needed to establish to what extent the light responses in other photoreceptors are the result of the summation of quantum bumps.

9.6 Summary

Psychophysical experiments on humans lead to the implication that rod photoreceptors produce a detectable signal when they absorb a single photon. Electrical recordings from both invertebrate and vertebrate photoreceptors demonstrate the existence of single-photon events, sometimes referred to as quantum bumps. There is evidence in some species that the entire photoresponse may result from the summation of these quantum bumps and that a change in bump size is a primary mechanism of adaptation. Further experiments are needed to establish the general validity of these observations.

10 Microphysiology of phototransduction

The absorption of a photon by a visual pigment is a highly localized event. Further insight into the phototransduction process can be obtained by investigating the actual spatial relationship between light absorption and conductance change in the plasma membrane.

10.1 Localization of excitation

The important problem of localization of excitation was initially investigated by Hagins and his colleagues first in squid and then in rat photoreceptors (Hagins et al., 1962; Hagins et al., 1970). They sectioned the eye in order to expose the whole length of the photoreceptors, and the cells were illuminated over a short section of their length as shown for the squid in Figure 10.1. They measured the extracellular voltage change produced by the extracellular currents that flow when the cells are stimulated by light. (Remember that the receptor potential results from a light-induced change in membrane ionic permeability.) In the squid, a light-induced permeability increase causes the cells to depolarize by allowing positive charge (primarily Na ions) to flow into the cells. This charge flowing into the cells can be detected as a current flowing in the extracellular space around the photoreceptors. They found that the inward current associated with the receptor potential was localized to an area very close to the site of illumination.

A similar approach was also used to study the spatial relationship between light absorption and excitation in rat rods (Hagins et al., 1970). Remember, in Chapter 7, we described how vertebrate photoreceptors respond to light with a membrane hyperpolarization that results primarily from a decrease in the membrane permeability to sodium. It turns out that this sodium permeability, which is suppressed by light, is mainly localized in the rod outer segment. The net result of this is that in the dark there is a steady, axially directed current flowing within and outside of every rod outer segment. The direction of this flow is such

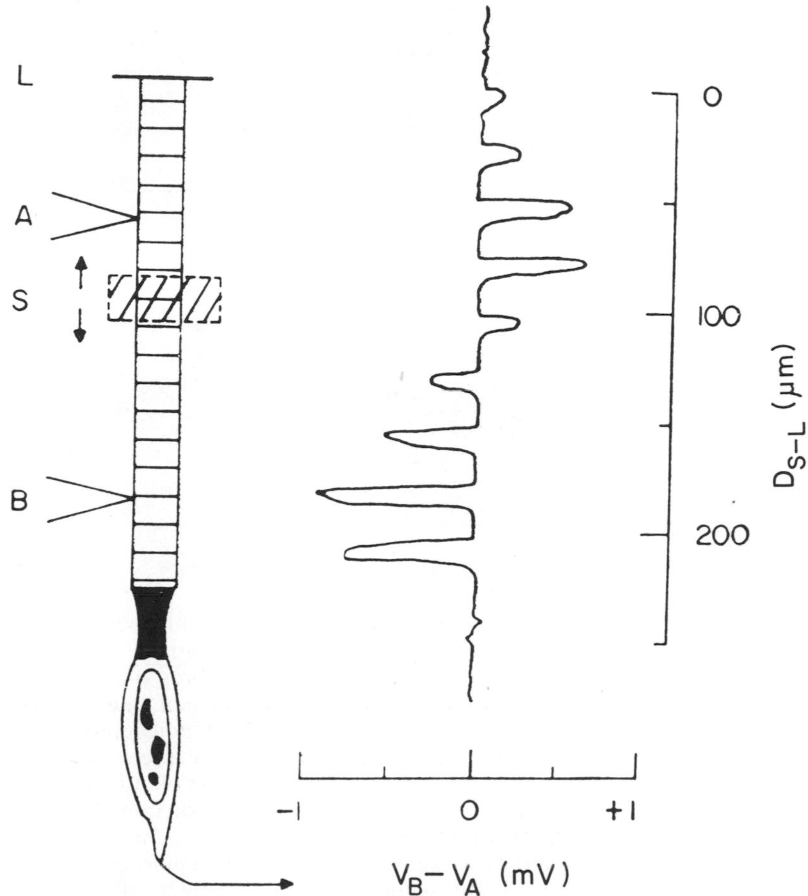

Figure 10.1. Extracellularly recorded potential around the distal segments in a retinal slice from a squid eye. The potential difference ($V_B - V_A$) was measured between two fixed micropipettes A and B. Photoreceptors were stimulated with light (S), which illuminated only a spatially confined region and which was moved along the length of the distal segments. The ordinate is the distance (D) between stimulus S and the internal limiting membrane L. The recorded potentials indicate that the light-induced current enters the photoreceptor in the region that is illuminated. (After Hagins et al., 1962.)

that a steady current, carried primarily by Na ions, enters the rod outer segment. An equal and opposite current flows out of the rod through its more proximal regions. The effect of light on the rod is to suppress locally this dark current.

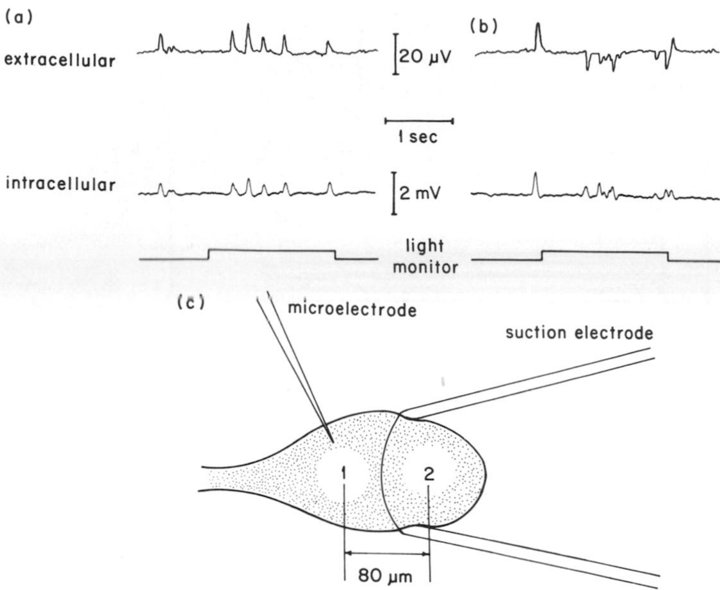

Figure 10.2. Local membrane currents associated with quantum bumps in a dark-adapted photoreceptor. (*c*) Schematized version of the recording situation showing the two stimulus spots labeled 1 and 2. In (*a*), the photoreceptor was stimulated at spot 1 and in (*b*), at spot 2. As shown in (*c*), a portion of a single photoreceptor is gently drawn into a glass suction electrode and a microelectrode is simultaneously inserted into the cell. Thus it is possible to measure simultaneously the extracellular currents using the suction electrode and the receptor transmembrane potential using the intracellular pipette. Two different regions of the photoreceptor, one inside, the other outside the suction electrode, could be stimulated with a small spot of light. In (*a*) and (*b*), the extracellularly recorded potential changes indicate that current enters the region of the photoreceptor that is illuminated by the spot of light. In all cases the receptor current depolarized the cell, which is shown by the intracellular recordings of the receptor transmembrane potential. Note the presence of spontaneous bumps preceding the light stimuli. (After Fein and Charlton, 1975*a*.)

Just as for the receptor potential, individual quantum bumps are also localized to the region of illumination. This measurement was accomplished by drawing a single *Limulus* photoreceptor into a suction electrode, as shown in Figure 10.2*c*, and thereby measuring the extracellular currents associated with only that particular photoreceptor (Fein and Charlton, 1975*a*). By this procedure, it was shown that the membrane current resulting from the absorption of individual quanta is

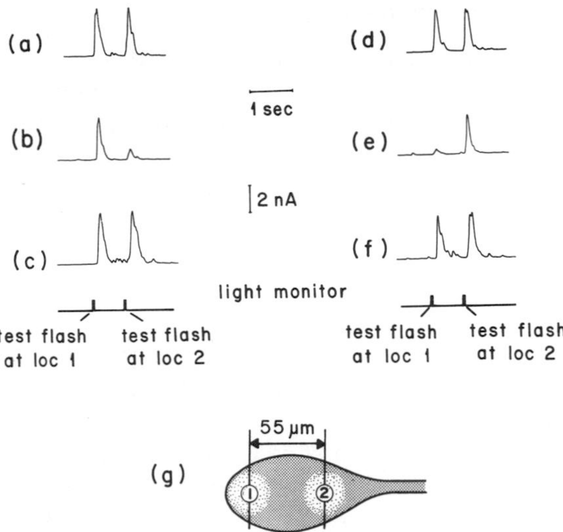

Figure 10.3. Localized desensitization produced by a spatially confined adapting light. (*a*)–(*f*) Responses of the photoreceptor recorded under voltage clamp; (*g*) schematized version of the photoreceptor, showing the two stimulus spots, labeled 1 and 2. Parts (*a*) and (*d*) show control responses elicited by the two spatially confined test flashes. Responses in (*b*) and (*e*) were recorded 2 sec after adapting stimuli at locations 2 and 1, respectively. (*e*) An adapting light at location 1 reduces the sensitivity only at 1, leaving the sensitivity at 2 nearly unaffected. (*b*) A similar localization of desensitization occurs if the adapting stimulus is positioned at 2. Parts (*c*) and (*f*) show that the receptor completely recovers from the adapting stimuli. (After Fein and Charlton, 1977*a*.)

localized to the region of absorption (see Figures 10.2*a* and *b*). The demonstration that individual quantum bumps are the result of a local membrane current strengthens the suggestion that the receptor potential results from a summation of these quantum bumps.

Thus, it has been clearly established that in both invertebrate and vertebrate photoreceptors excitation is spatially localized to the region of photon absorption. These experiments should not be taken to imply that excitation does not spread at all beyond the site of photon absorption. Rather, they give an upper limit for its spread, this upper limit being not more than about 10 μm. The actual spread may be less: other evidence to be discussed in Chapter 11 indicates that the extent of the spread is closer to a few microns.

10.2 Localization of adaptation

Given that excitation is spatially localized, it is natural to enquire whether adaptation is similarly constrained. Hagins et al. (1962) first investigated this possibility and reported that adaptation in squid photoreceptors was localized to an area close to the site where the light was absorbed. Subsequently, the localization of adaptation was quantitatively investigated in *Limulus* ventral photoreceptors (Fein and Charlton, 1975*b*), as is illustrated in Figure 10.3. Although adaptation is localized in ventral photoreceptors, there were clear indications that adaptation spreads beyond the region of illumination, and this spread could not be explained by light scatter. Thus, the physical change that is responsible for adaptation must spread somewhat beyond the region where the light is absorbed.

Fein and Charlton (1975*b*) also showed that the reduction of bump size attributable to adaptation was also similarly localized. A direct demonstration of local adaptation in a vertebrate photoreceptor using the suction–electrode technique has recently been reported by Jagger (1979), indicating that localized adaptation is a property of both vertebrate and invertebrate photoreceptors. This was independently confirmed by McNaughton et al. (1980), who showed that, in the toad, the spatial spread is about 8 μm for both excitation and adaptation.

10.3 Summary

Local excitation and adaptation of invertebrate and vertebrate photoreceptors has been demonstrated in those few preparations where it has been technically feasible. The individual quantum bumps that have been suggested to make up the photoresponse have been shown to arise near the region of illumination and to suffer a localized reduction in amplitude. Some aspect of the molecular events involved in excitation and adaptation must be responsible for the spatial localization of these phenomena. Any proposed model for excitation and/or adaptation must be able to account for the spatial localization of these processes.

11 Molecular mechanisms of excitation

One obvious question that arises from the physiological findings discussed in the previous chapters is: How does the absorption of light by the visual pigment molecules bring about the change in membrane ionic permeability? The answer to this question still eludes us. At this time, however, many scientists are actively in search of the answer. What we shall attempt to do in this chapter is to give a brief review of the current approaches that are being taken to resolve this issue.

11.1 Constraints for any molecular model

Before discussing any particular models, it will be instructive to review the requirements that the physiological findings place upon any potential model.

11.1.1 Action at a distance

The need for action at a distance is a salient feature of excitation. This requirement stems from the finding that excitation spreads from the point of photon absorption over a considerable area of photoreceptor membrane. One of the most striking pieces of evidence to indicate that excitation spreads is the finding that it takes relatively few photoactivated rhodopsins to activate the available ionic channels completely. For example, in the toad rod, a single photoisomerization anywhere in the outer segment suppresses the dark current by about 3% (Baylor et al., 1979*a*, *b*). Irrespective of how uniformly the Na channels are distributed along the plasma membrane, a 3% decrease in dark current requires that excitation spreads over at least 3% of the plasma membrane. In the *Limulus* ventral photoreceptor, one photoactivated rhodopsin can activate about 0.3% of the total light-activated current (Brown and Coles, 1979). The requirement for action at a distance is also demanded by the structure of vertebrate rods. Most of the visual pigment of rods is located in the rod disk membrane, and it is the Na permeability of the plasma membrane that is regulated by light (see Chapter 7). It has been convincingly demonstrated that most of the rod disks are not continuous with the plasma membrane (see Cohen, 1972). Yet the absolute sensitivity of rods requires that the absorption of light by rhodopsin located in the disks must be able to excite the rods. These observations require that an excitatory signal must spread from the disk membrane to the plasma membrane. The characteristics of the bumps (single-photon events; see Chapter 9) of *Limulus* ventral photoreceptors also indicate the need for action at a distance. The conductance increase associated with a bump can be as large as 10,000 to 50,000 pS. Because a single channel has a conductance of about 20 pS (Wong, 1978), the absorption of a single photon opens approximately 1000 ionic channels. This clearly requires an excitatory signal to spread from the site of photon absorption. The inescapable conclusion of these observations is that action at a distance is an obligatory component of excitation. This requirement strongly implies the involvement of a diffusible cytoplasmic transmitter in transduction. Based on the studies cited in this paragraph, we can estimate that excitation spreads several micrometers from the site of photon absorption.

11.1.2 Single-photon sensitivity

Perhaps the most striking requirement of visual excitation is its sensitivity to single photons (see Chapter 9). Any chemical or physical change that is believed to be involved in excitation must exhibit the required sensitivity to single photons. The detectability of single photons leads to the following simple quantitative analysis. Because the data of the previous section suggest the involvement of a diffusible transmitter substance, let us suppose that excitation changes the cytoplasmic concentration of the transmitter molecules near the region of excitation; say that N molecules of this substance are present in the region where excitation occurs. We know that the absorption of a single photon must lead to a detectable change in the number of these molecules. Because of random motion due to thermal energy, the actual number of molecules present in a given volume will vary with time. Typically, this variation about the mean is approximately equal to the square root of the mean, or, in our case, $N^{1/2}$. In order for a single photon to produce a detectable signal, it would have to cause a change in the number of our hypothetical molecules that is at least as great as their inherent variability. Thus, if there were nominally N molecules present, a single photon would have to change the number of molecules by at least $N^{1/2}$. If there were only 100 molecules of our hypothetical substance present, one photon would have changed the number of molecules by 10 molecules, or 10%. If there were 10^6 molecules, the required change would be 1000 molecules, or 0.1%. Thus, depending on the resting level of our hypothetical substance, the requirement for the number of molecules turned over (increased or decreased) per photon will vary.

11.1.3 Intensity–response curve

Any model for excitation must generate the relationship between light intensity and receptor response discussed in Section 8.2.1. The basic requirements are that the transduction process be initially linear with light intensity and subsequently saturated. Various processes meet these requirements and can give rise to the relationship described by Equation (8.1).

11.1.4 Temporal requirements of excitation

Not to be overlooked are the temporal requirements of excitation. For both invertebrate and vertebrate photoreceptors, there is a latent period between the absorption of light by the visual pigment molecule and the occurrence of the photoresponse. A very rough estimate for the latent period of the response to a brief dim flash for a dark-adapted photoreceptor is about 100 msec [see Table 3 in the review by Hagins (1972)]. Under these conditions, the duration of the light response is roughly 1 sec. The latency and duration of the response vary quantitatively with the intensity and duration of the light stimulus.

11.2 Internal transmitter model for visual excitation

All the requirements previously given can, in principle, be satisfied by the internal transmitter model just cited and are equally met whether or not light causes an increase or a decrease in the transmitter's cytoplasmic concentration. For light to increase cytoplasmic concentration, the absorption of light should cause the release and (or) the production of the transmitter. The presence of the transmitter gives rise in some way to the permeability change. Termination of the light response results from uptake and (or) degradation of the transmitter. For light to decrease cytoplasmic concentration, it should destroy and (or) stimulate the sequesterization of a transmitter that already preexists in the cytoplasm. The idea of an internal transmitter is not recent (for example, see Fuortes and Hodgkin, 1964; Borsellino and Fuortes, 1968; Baylor and Fuortes, 1970). Cone (1973) provides a thorough discussion of the need for an internal transmitter in both vertebrate and invertebrate photoreceptors. It should be stressed that, aside from nature's tendency to conserve molecular mechanisms for similar cellular functions, there is no a priori reason why the same transmitter should mediate excitation in all photoreceptors. In fact, the currently available evidence, which will be discussed next, indicates that the putative transmitters of vertebrates and some invertebrates may be different; similar exceptions could just as well exist among vertebrates.

11.3 Criteria to be met by a transmitter

There are two fundamental tests that any substance suspected of being directly involved in photoreceptor excitation must meet. It is necessary to show that a change in the concentration of the putative substance is both necessary and sufficient to produce photoreceptor excitation. Most tests of any particular substance fall into two categories, physiological and chemical. The physiological tests revolve around showing identity of action. In this type of test, application of the substance to the photoreceptor must be shown to mimic quantitatively the effects of light. The chemical tests involve showing that changes in the concentration of the putative substance actually occur as the result of light. These concentration changes must demonstrate the appropriate absolute sensitivity to single photons and the correct temporal characteristics.

In 1958, Paton proposed a set of criteria to be satisfied by a substance before it can be considered to be a true transmitter. Though the formulations were originally made with synaptic transmitters in mind, they have a general validity for all types of transmitters. In the context of our discussion, it is worthwhile to restate Paton's criteria.

1. Criterion for transmitter presence: Transmitter should exist in sufficient amounts in the receptor or compartment from which it is released.
2. Criterion for light effect on transmitter concentration: Light should alter transmitter's concentration within the cytoplasm and, if released from somewhere, also within stated compartment.
3. Criterion for identity of action for an artificially caused change in concentration: Varying the transmitter's concentration in the dark should mimic the effect of light.
4. Criterion for the effect of modifiers: Application of blocking or enhancing agents should equally effect both the light- and artificially induced responses.

5. Criterion for the necessary enzymes: The receptor or its compartment must possess the necessary enzymes for the light effect.

11.4 Hydrogen ions as the internal transmitter

Because bacteriorhodopsin functions as a light-activated proton pump (see Chapter 4) and because proton movements are involved in the interconversion of metarhodopsins (see visual cycles in Chapter 6), hydrogen ions might play a role in visual excitation. Only two of Paton's criteria have so far been tested – the identity of action of an artificially evoked pH change and the effect of agents that suppress alterations in pH – and the proton hypothesis has failed by both criteria.

Coles and Brown (1976) injected *Limulus* ventral photoreceptors with a variety of pH buffers. The idea was to suppress any light-induced changes in intracellular pH. They found that a change in intracellular pH buffering capacity had only a small effect on the latency of the photoresponse. From these findings, they concluded that excitation of the photoreceptor is probably not mediated by a change in intracellular pH.

During the metarhodopsin I → metarhodopsin II reaction, protons are taken up by vertebrate rhodopsin (see Section 6.4). In a weakly buffered system, this proton uptake can lead to an alkaline pH change, which can be artificially induced by exposing cells to a perfusate containing NH_3/NH_4^+. When rods of the toad or axolotl were exposed to a perfusate that contained NH_3/NH_4^+, the membrane depolarized and, hence, did not mimic the hyperpolarization observed upon illumination (Pinto and Ostroy, 1978). Thus, it appears *unlikely* that a change in pH_i mediates the light response of rods.

Taken together, the foregoing evidence indicates that the biological activity of the visual pigments of vertebrates and invertebrates is different from that of bacteriorhodopsin and, more importantly, protons are unlikely to be the internal transmitter.

11.5 Calcium as the internal transmitter

11.5.1 Invertebrate photoreceptors

As mentioned in Chapter 7, the photoreceptors of the distal retina of the scallop hyperpolarize in light (Gorman and McReynolds, 1969; McReynolds and Gorman, 1970*a*). The reversal potential of the photoresponse and ionic substitution experiments suggest that light makes the cell permeable to K (McReynolds and Gorman, 1970*b*; Gorman and McReynolds, 1974). McReynolds and Gorman (1974) found that metabolic inhibitors caused a rapid hyperpolarization and increase in membrane permeability, similar to the effect of light. They suggested that the effects of the metabolic inhibitors were due to an increase in intracellular Ca concentration, raising the possibility that the photoresponse may also be due to a change in intracellular Ca. None of Paton's criteria have yet been rigorously tested for this hypothesis.

Light has been found to alter the membrane potential of certain large neurons within the ganglia of invertebrates (Arvanitaki and Chalazonitis, 1961). These neurons do not appear to be photoreceptors in the conventional sense in that they do not contain rhodopsin and are relatively insensitive to light (Baur et al., 1977; Andersen and Brown, 1979). They will be discussed, however, because they represent a well-characterized system. Illumination of an *Aplysia* giant neuron evokes a membrane hyperpolarization that results from an increase in K permeability. The response was suggested to result from a light-activated increase in intracellular Ca, which, in turn, increases K permeability (Brown and Brown, 1973). Injection of Ca into the neuron was found to hyperpolarize the cell, and injection of EGTA (a Ca buffer) abolished or greatly reduced the light response. Such findings partly satisfy criteria 3 and 4. Illumination of *Aplysia* neurons causes their pigmented organelles, the lipochondria, to undergo ultrastructural changes and to release Ca. It has been suggested that the lipochondria are the intracellular site of photopigment and are the source of Ca that gives rise to the photoresponse (Baur et al., 1977). If this were the case, then diffusion of Ca from the lipochondria to the plasma membrane might determine the temporal characteristics of the light response. Theoretical analysis by Andersen et al. (1979) indicates that, indeed, diffusion can adequately account for the experimentally observed response wave form. These experiments satisfy criterion 1 and partly satisfy criterion 2. Attempts to detect a light-induced rise in intracellular Ca have so far met with failure (Owen and Brown, 1980). At the time of this writing, criterion 5 had not yet been tested for these light-sensitive neurons.

11.5.2 Vertebrate photoreceptors

The first report for calcium's role as a putative transmitter in vertebrate receptors is due to Yoshikami and Hagins (1971), who observed that in rat rods elevation of extracellular Ca qualitatively mimicked the effect of light, that is, Ca suppressed the dark current. Based on their important, albeit limited, observations, they hypothesized that a light-induced rise in intracellular Ca decreases the Na permeability of the outer segment, thereby giving rise to the light response. Their reasonable assumption was that increased extracellular Ca leads to Ca influx into the cell, resulting in an increased cytoplasmic level. Although they had no evidence for the identity of the storage compartment from which light-initiated Ca release could occur, it was reasonable for them to hypothesize that the source was the intradiskal space because vertebrate outer segments contain no other membrane-bound organelles. This then is the Ca hypothesis for excitation of vertebrate rods and cones.

Because calcium is one of the best candidates for the intracellular transmitter, the experimental data for each of Paton's criteria will be individually considered.

Criterion 1. Sufficient Ca within disks. Statistical noise analysis, which was discussed earlier in Section 11.1.2 predicts that on the order of 100 Ca ions must be released into the cytoplasm at threshold. The same conclusion can be derived from more rigorous mathematical considerations (Cone, 1973). Each disk in a frog rod contains about 10^5 Ca ions, equivalent to a total concentration of about 5 mM (Szuts and Conc, 1977). This amount appears to be a sufficiently large reservoir to sustain release even for saturating light flashes where, on the average, one out of every ten disks absorbs a photon. For cones, the normal 1-mM extracellular Ca concentration provides a nearly inexhaustible supply of Ca for release into the intracellular compartment. Thus, this criterion must be considered to be satisfied.

Criterion 2. Light effects on cytoplasmic and intradiskal Ca. The only evidence yet obtained for a rise in cytoplasmic Ca is the recent report that in excised living retinas illumination increases Ca concentration in the interstitial space around rod outer segments (Gold and Korenbrot, 1980; Yoshikami et al., 1980). Presumably the increase is due to an efflux resulting from an initial rise in cytoplasmic Ca rather than just a direct activation of pumping rate or suppression of a continual influx in the dark. Unfortunately, light-induced Ca release from disks, which is the most direct test of the Ca hypothesis, has repeatedly failed to be observed (Szuts and Cone, 1977; Liebman, 1978). There is no evidence that even under physiological conditions such light-induced fluxes occur (Szuts, 1980). However, some insignificantly small light-induced Ca release can be recorded if disks are initially sonicated (Smith et al., 1977). On the basis of indirect evidence, this criterion must be considered to have been satisfied only partially.

Criterion 3. The identity of action of exogenously applied Ca. In both rods and cones, the dark current diminishes and finally disappears as the external calcium concentration is raised to 20 mM (Hagins, 1972). The effects of high extracellular Ca and a background light on the flash response of turtle cones and toad rods have been carefully studied by Bertrand et al. (1978) and Bastian and Fain (1979). Both sets of investigators found that, under conditions where background light and elevated extracellular Ca produce equal membrane hyperpolarizations, the changes induced by the two procedures on response to flashes were entirely different. Hence it may be that high external Ca mimics light in that it blocks the light-sensitive permeability, but it differs in other important aspects from the effects of light. Moreover, it is not clear in these experiments whether high external Ca acts directly on the outside of the cell membrane or has an internal site of action.

Treating rods with the chemical X537A (which increases membrane permeability to Ca as well as other divalent and monovalent cations) reduces the concentration of Ca in the bathing solution needed to suppress the dark current, causes membrane hyperpolarization, and suppresses the light response (Hagins and Yoshikami, 1974; Bastian and Fain, 1979). These experiments indicate that an increase in intracellular Ca activity will suppress the dark current and hyperpolarize the photoreceptor. In a related experiment, Brown et al. (1977*a*) found that iontophoretic injection of Ca into a rod results in a hyperpolarization that decays with a time course similar to the decay of the receptor potential.

Taken as a whole, these results indicate that an increase in intracellular Ca will partially mimic light by suppressing the Na permeability of the outer segment.

Criterion 4. Removal of calcium, with or without the use of Ca-chelating agents. Exposing rods to below normal Ca increases the dark current and causes the membrane to depolarize while the amplitude of the light response increases greatly (Yoshikami and Hagins, 1972; Brown and Pinto, 1974; Lipton et al., 1977*a*; Yau et al., 1981). This can be explained by an increase in the light-dependent permeability in darkness. On prolonged exposure to below normal Ca, desensitization of the light response occurs (Yoshikami and Hagins, 1972; Lipton et al., 1977*a*). Presumably decreasing the extracellular Ca depletes the rods of their internal stores of Ca.

Certain physiological tests of the Ca hypothesis are simpler in cones than in rods because in cones the presumptive source of calcium is the extracellular solution. One of the more important tests of the hypothesis is to reduce greatly the extracellular Ca and thereby lower the source of calcium available for excitation. This type of experiment has been performed in the cones of the turtle (Bertrand et al., 1978), pigeon (Arden and Low, 1978), and lizard (Yoshikami and Hagins, 1978) using the calcium buffer EGTA to reduce the extracellular Ca. The results of these three studies have led to conflicting conclusions. The authors of the first two studies concluded that extracellular Ca was not the source of the internal transmitter, whereas the third study was interpreted as being consistent with the original hypothesis. Obviously, further work is needed to settle this point.

The introduction of a Ca buffer into rods reduces the photoresponse to dim flashes (Hagins and Yoshikami, 1977; Brown et al., 1977*a*). Presumably, the desensitization results because the Ca buffer binds some of the Ca that is released on illumination, thereby suppressing the resultant permeability decrease. The injection of EGTA into a rod results in depolarization (Brown et al., 1977*a*). This can be explained if EGTA lowers the intracellular Ca concentration, thereby increasing the permeability of Na in darkness.

To summarize the implications of these findings, it would appear that a rise in intracellular Ca is a necessary step for rod excitation. On the basis of the available data, the same cannot be said for cones.

Criterion 5. Presence of enzymes to regulate free calcium. As with light-induced Ca release, no convincing evidence has yet been given to show that disks actively accumulate Ca (Szuts, 1980). It appears that rod disks lack both the required Ca-releasing and Ca-accumulating properties.

A review of the evidence. As originally stated, the Ca hypothesis was meant to encompass excitation in both rods and cones. For a variety of reasons, the hypothesis has been tested much more extensively in rods than in cones. Criteria 2 and 5 have not been tested for cones, and tests of criterion 4 have led to conflicting results. Criterion 1 has been completely and criterion 3 partially satisfied. On the basis of the present evidence, there is not much support for the Ca hypothesis in cones.

The evidence is much more favorable for rods: criterion 1 is fully and criteria 2, 3, and 4 are at least partially satisfied, with positive evidence lacking only for criterion 5. Unfortunately, the failure to demonstrate any light-induced Ca release or uptake from rod disks has put the entire Ca hypothesis into disrepute (Fatt, 1979) even though on the basis of other criteria, it at least partially meets the test. At this writing, Ca still remains the most promising of the putative transmitters. The Ca hypothesis could be retained if the light-sensitive source of Ca were not the internal space of disks. Perhaps some bound form of Ca within the cytoplasm could be the long-sought source.

11.6 cGMP as the internal transmitter

Cyclic nucleotides are ubiquitous cellular substances and perform an important role in regulating enzymes. Their possible importance in receptors was first heralded in a report by Bitensky et al. (1971). Although the report eventually turned out to be wrong in certain details, it correctly emphasized the potential importance of cyclic nucleotides. It initiated a series of experiments by many investigators that eventually led to the proposal for guanosine 3′5′-cyclic-monophosphate (cGMP) being the intracellular transmitter. The cGMP hypothesis rested on the observation that light destroys cGMP within rod cytoplasm. The reduction of the cGMP concentration was sufficiently large and occurred sufficiently fast to be a potential modifier of Na channels.

Cyclic GMP is formed from guanosine 5′-triphosphate (GTP) by the enzyme guanylate cyclase and is hydrolyzed to guanosine 5′-monophosphate (GMP) by the enzyme phosphodiesterase (PDE). The action of light is on the degradative pathway (phosphodiesterase) rather than the synthetic pathway (guanylate cyclase).

As was done for Ca, we shall review the experimental evidence to see whether or not cGMP satisfies Paton's criteria.

Criterion 1. Presence of cGMP within cytoplasm. Direct measurements have established that cGMP exists in all photoreceptors in which it has been sought. In vertebrate rod outer segments, the basal concentration is on the order of 30 μM, or about 10^7 molecules (Woodruff and Bownds, 1979). The molecule's concentration may be an order of magnitude less in other receptors such as cones (Farber et al., 1981) or *Limulus* ventral photoreceptors (Schmidt and Farber, 1980).

Criterion 2. Light effects on cytoplasmic cGMP levels. Three types of preparations have typically been used to study the effects of light on the level of cGMP in rods: (a) excised living retinas, (b) isolated, but otherwise intact, outer segments, and (c) isolated, fragmented outer segments. (a) In the excised frog retina, cGMP levels were not significantly reduced 1 sec after illumination; significant decreases were detected only 3 to 5 sec after the stimulus (Goridis et al, 1977; Kilbride and Ebrey, 1979; Govardovskii and Berman, 1981). This rate of change is not rapid enough to be involved in excitation. To close Na channels, cGMP concentrations should decrease within the latency of the photoresponse, that is, within 100 msec. It could be argued that only a small fraction of the total retinal cGMP is in a compartment that is functionally active during excitation. Measurements of retinal cGMP levels might not be sensitive enough to detect small changes in the content of cGMP in this compartment. (b) Bleaching 1% of the rhodopsin in isolated outer segments with intact plasma membranes produced no detectable change in cGMP levels within 10 to 60 sec according to Robinson and Hagins (1980). On the other hand, Woodruff et al. (1977) reported that bleaching one rhodopsin molecule can lead to the hydrolysis of 1000 to 2000 molecules of cGMP within a fraction of a second. The magnitude of this decrease is just barely a sufficiently large signal from statistical noise analysis. Remember that in the dark there are about 10^7 cGMP molecules. The light effect should exceed the thermal variability, which is $10^{7/2}$, or about 3×10^3. The reason why only some and not all investigators see the light effect is probably due to the physiological state of the isolated outer segments and to the effects of Ca on the hydrolysis reaction (Polans et al., 1981). (c) Using fragmented outer segments, Yee and Liebman (1978) found that proton release accompanying cGMP hydrolysis could be detected within 100 msec following a bright flash.

In conclusion, it seems reasonable that it has yet to be convincingly established that in intact rods decreases in cGMP levels are of sufficient magnitude and occur rapidly enough to be involved in excitation.

Criterion 3. Identity of action of exogenously applied cGMP. Because illumination leads to the destruction and not to the synthesis of cGMP, exogenous application of the molecule should not mimic light. One might predict that cGMP injection would depolarize rods because the excess cGMP might result in more Na channels being open than are normally open in the dark. Such a depolarization resulting from cGMP injection does in fact occur (Miller and Nicol, 1979; Brown and Waloga, 1981). Moreover, the amplitude of the light response increases during the depolarization following cGMP injection, suggesting that light can close the Na channels presumably opened by excess cGMP injection. Superficially, these findings appear to be consistent with the notion that a light-induced decrease in intracellular cGMP levels is involved in excitation. On the other hand, such an interpretation is at odds with the results of preliminary experiments using 8-Bromo-cGMP, an hydrolysis resistant analog of cGMP (Waloga and Bitensky, 1981). Because intracellular injection of 8-Bromo-cGMP depolarized the membrane of toad rods and also increased the response amplitude just as cGMP did, hydrolysis of cGMP does not appear to be an obligatory step in the process of visual excitation. All these results do, however, support the notion that cGMP is an important factor in determining the membrane potential and the light response of rods.

Criterion 4. Effects of inhibitors of cGMP metabolism. Pharmacological agents that block the degradation of cGMP by the enzyme phosphodiesterase have been thoroughly investigated. For example, it was found that exposure of rods to isobutylmethylxanthine (IBMX), a PDE inhibitor, depolarized the membrane of rods and increased their light response (Lipton et al., 1977*b*; Brown and Waloga, 1981). These results are the same as with cGMP injection (and in fact they should be because PDE inhibitors in effect increase cytoplasmic cGMP levels) and are also subject to the same criticism: an increase in the light response is not what one would expect if activation of PDE were directly involved in excitation.

Criterion 5. Enzymes for cGMP metabolism. In contrast with the Ca hypothesis, the evidence for the existence of the required metabolic enzymes for cGMP is overwhelming. Historically, these enzymes were discovered before the level of cGMP was actually measured within receptors. The extensive work with these enzymes formed the groundwork on which the cGMP hypothesis was based.

As in all cells in nature, cGMP in photoreceptors is synthesized from GTP via a single reaction and is similarly degraded via a single reaction to GMP. Synthesis is catalyzed by the enzyme guanylate cyclase, and degradation by the enzyme phosphodiesterase. The reactions are as follows:

$$\text{GTP} \xrightarrow{\text{cyclase}} \text{cGMP} \xrightarrow{\text{PDE}} \text{GMP}$$
$$+$$
$$\text{pyrophosphate}$$

Within rods the concentration of GTP is about 1 to 2 mM and GMP is about 0.5 mM (Robinson and Hagins, 1979) and, as previously mentioned, the concentration of cGMP is about 30 μM. It should be noted that the above enzymes can also use the adenyl analogs (ATP, cAMP) as substrates, but in rods they prefer to interact with the guanyl nucleotides. As indicated, the action of light is on the degradative pathway (phosphodiesterase) rather than the synthetic pathway (guanylate cyclase). Phosphodiesterase can be removed from the photoreceptor membrane and purified (Miki et al., 1975), which suggests that it is a separate molecule from rhodopsin. The experiments of Keirns et al. (1975) indicate that the first step in the activation of phosphodiesterase is the absorption of light by rhodopsin. They reported also that half-maximal activation of phosphodiesterase occurs when only 0.05% of the rhodopsin has been bleached. More recent measurements indicate that PDE is 50% activated by bleaching 1 rhodopsin in 80,000 (Yee and Liebman, 1978).

A review of the evidence. Taken together, the findings cited under criteria 1, 2, and 5 unequivocally establish that cGMP metabolism is an important and active constituent of rod biochemistry. Alterations in the cGMP content of rods effect both the receptor's transmembrane potential and its light response (criteria 3 and 4). Nevertheless, in terms of the original question being considered in this section, we are led to conclude that a light-activated hydrolysis of cGMP does not appear to be an obligatory component of receptor excitation. This conclusion should not be taken to imply that cGMP metabolism plays no role in transduction. Rather, to the contrary, we believe that future work will elucidate an important role for cGMP metabolism in rod excitation or possibly adaptation.

11.7 The physiological function of light-activated rhodopsin

Now that we have cited the putative intracellular transmitters, we shall once again return to the question raised in Chapter 6: What is the physiological function of light-activated rhodopsin molecules? Of course, the answer partly depends on the identity of the intracellular transmitter. For instance, the initial formulation of the Ca hypothesis requires that photoactivated rhodopsin either directly or indirectly opens Ca channels through the membrane in which it is embedded. This could be accomplished in an elegant way if the molecule itself were a Ca channel. Then light absorption would just simply transform it from a closed to an open state. However, existing biochemical evidence does not support this notion.

Though cGMP hydrolysis may not be the causal factor that directly modulates the state of Na channels, the biochemical evidence for the interaction of light-activated rhodopsin and the previously described phosphodiesterase is overwhelming. Most of this evidence is based on data from rod disks because the amount of purified rod outer segments is appropriately large for such biochemical studies.

Three proteins in addition to rhodopsin have been implicated in the regulation of phosphodiesterase activity by light. These are illustrated in Figure 11.1. The three proteins include the aforementioned phosphodiesterase (mol wt. 240,000; Miki et al., 1975) a nucleotide-binding protein, commonly abbreviated as *N*-protein (mol wt. 39,000; Fung et al., 1981) and a "helper" protein (*H*), necessary for the function of the *N*-protein (mol wt. 60,000; Shinozawa et al., 1980). In the inactive form

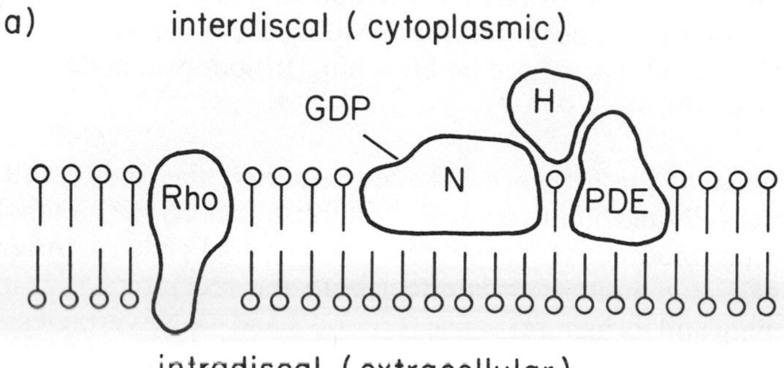

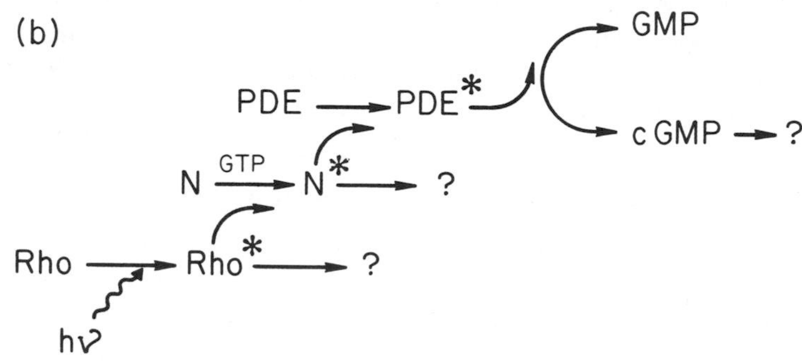

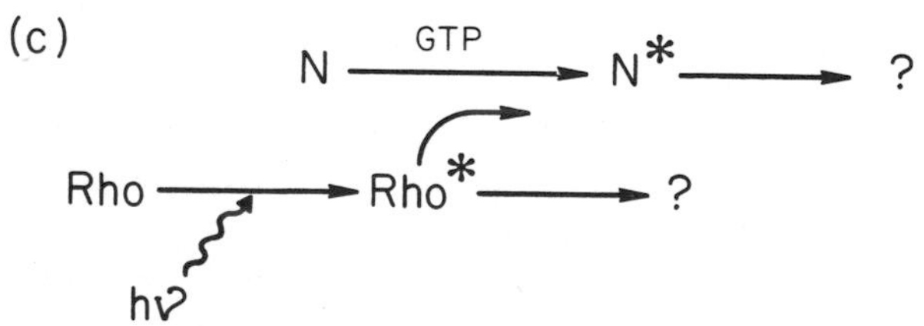

Figure 11.1. Early light-activated enzymatic steps within photoreceptors. (*a*) Protein components of rod disk involved in regulation of phosphodiesterase. These are Rho = rhodopsin, *N* = nucleotide-binding protein, *H* = helper protein, PDE = phosphodiesterase (see text for a more detailed description of these proteins). (*b*) Reactions initiated by photoactivated rhodopsin in vertebrate rods. (*c*) Reactions initiated by photoactivated rhodopsin in *Limulus* ventral photoreceptors. The asterisk represents the activated form of the stated proteins. One of these early steps eventually leads to a change in the Na-permeability of the plasma membrane. The question marks in (*b*) and (*c*) are meant to indicate as yet unknown reactions that may be involved in transduction.

that eixsts in the dark, the *N*-protein contains a tightly bound guanosine 5′-diphosphate (GDP). On light activation, it undergoes a sequence of reactions: it exchanges the bound GDP for GTP, activates the PDE, and, with the assistance of the *H*-protein, hydrolyzes GTP at its terminal phosphate, thereby returning to the inactive state. The resulting GDP remains tightly bound to *N*. The *N*-protein is extremely sensitive to light: Half-maximal activation occurs when on the order of 1 out of every 3000 rhodopsins is photoactivated (Wheeler and Bitensky, 1977; Fung and Stryer, 1980). In addition, it is an obligatory intermediary in the light-activation of PDE (Shinozawa et al., 1979; Fung et al., 1981). The PDE, *N*, and *H* are peripheral membrane proteins that are only loosely associated with the disk. It is not yet clear what fraction of these proteins is actually on the disk membrane under physiological conditions. They may be cytoplasmic-soluble components that depend on a dynamic interaction with the disks membrane. Even when membrane bound, they are less abundant than rhodopsin. For example, the molar ratio of PDE to rhodopsin is approximately 1 to 900 (Miki et al., 1975).

Based on the evidence just given, it appears that at least in rod disks one function (enzymatic) of light-activated rhodopsin is to activate the nucleotide-binding protein. Provided that GTP is available, the *N*-protein is transformed into an active state, which in turn stimulates the phosphodiesterase to split cGMP. This cascade of enzymatic reactions is illustrated in Figure 11.1. Though the involved proteins are not equally concentrated within the disks, lateral diffusion within the membrane (and cytoplasm?) apparently makes interaction between them possible. A single photoactivated rhodopsin appears to activate as many as 500 *N*-proteins, each of which is then able to interact with many PDEs. Recent pharmacological evidence strongly suggests that the activation of an *N*-protein (Figure 11.1) apparently also occurs in at least some invertebrates (Fein and Corson, 1981). Injection of known specific activators of the *N*-protein into *Limulus* ventral photoreceptors leads to discrete waves in the dark that are similar to quantum bumps. Thus, it appears that the coupling of the visual pigment to an *N*-protein may be a common feature of all photoreceptors and may possibly be the physiological function of photoactivated rhodopsin.

As Pober and Bitensky (1979) remarked, a number of similarities exist between the light-activated PDE of rods and hormone-sensitive adenylate cyclase systems. In both cases, the external stimulus (hormone or light) activates a membrane-bound receptor molecule, which in turn stimulates the activity of a nucleotide-binding protein. The activated form of this *N*-protein then activates a third protein, which happens to be PDE in rods and adenylate cyclase in most hormone systems. The obvious conclusion is that rhodopsin essentially behaves as a hormone receptor: *its enzymatic function is to activate a nucleotide-binding protein.* The universality and correctness of this homology awaits experimental verification.

11.8 Identity of physiologically active form of rhodopsin

It is not yet known what subtle changes must occur in the chemical structure of rhodopsin to lead to excitation or to the stimulation of *N*-protein. Nor is the lifetime of the active form known. One entertaining notion is that rhodopsin's physiologically active form correlates with one of the photochemical intermediates. Any photoproduct that has either formed or decayed within the latent period of the light response is a potential candidate. In vertebrate photoreceptors, the 100-msec latency is sufficiently long to encompass all the intermediates preceding and including meta II rhodopsin. Similarly, all the intermediates up to metarhodopsin are potential candidates in invertebrates. Unfortunately, it is not known which, if any, photointermediates correspond to the physiologically active form. What is known is that neither the formation nor the decay of any photointermediate is the rate-limiting reaction of phototransduction (Hagins, 1972). Although this does not rule out a one-to-one correspondence, it should be stated that there is no a priori reason why such correlation should occur. The physiologically active site may be sufficiently far removed from the chromophore-binding site so that aside from the initial phototrigger the two regions of the molecule may be ''uncoupled'' from each other.

11.9 Quantitative models of photoreceptor excitation

Hodgkin and his colleagues succeeded in providing quantitative models of photoreceptor excitation and adaptation for both invertebrate and vertebrate photoreceptors (Fuortes and Hodgkin, 1964; Baylor et al., 1974). These models successfully describe the quantitative aspect of the photoresponse for both short- and long-duration light stimuli and provide useful descriptions for excitation and adaptation. Unfortunately, their usefulness in understanding the physiological reactions has been limited for several reasons. First, various physical processes can generate the types of mathematical equations that were set forth [see discussions in Levinson (1972) and Hagins (1972)]. Second, the parameters used in the models are not uniquely determined, so that a variety of models could fit the experimental data equally well. Third, at present, experimenters have been unable to measure any processes in the photoreceptor that correlate with parameters in the models. This does not mean, however, that these models are without their use. Having a quantitative kinetic description of the photoresponse has proved useful for comparing the photoresponse with visual pigment kinetics (see Hagins, 1972). Also, it has been shown that there is a quantitative relationship between the changes in sensitivity and time scale of the photoresponse that occur with light adaptation in both invertebrate (Fuortes and Hodgkin, 1964) and vertebrate (Baylor and Hodgkin, 1974) photoreceptors.

11.10 Summary

A number of chemical changes, among them the activation of the enzyme phosphodiesterase, occur as the result of the absorption of light by rhodopsin. At present, there is little physiological evidence to indicate what role these chemical changes play in phototransduction. On the other hand, there is ample physiological evidence to suggest a role for Ca ions in the excitation of both vertebrate and some invertebrate photoreceptors.

12 Molecular models of adaptation

In the last chapter, we presented the current evidence on the molecular mechanism of receptor excitation, and in this chapter we shall do the same for adaptation. The molecular aspects of adaptation may be just as, if not more, complicated to unravel than those of excitation. We certainly know less about them. We do know, however, that a simple explanation, such as the notion that sensitivity goes simply as the inverse of the number of rhodopsin molecules that have not yet been photoactivated (Section 8.2.4), is inconsistent with experimental observations.

Whenever adaptation is discussed, it is important to keep in mind the distinction between the two types: light and dark adaptation. As mentioned in Section 8.2.3, these two processes are not simply the reverse of each other. Therefore, experimental evidence obtained from one type cannot necessarily be applied to the other. Our understanding of the molecular mechanisms of adaptation often rests on what happens during light adaptation, and accordingly, this aspect will receive more emphasis in the ensuing discussion.

12.1 Constraints for any molecular model

Before considering any particular model, it is worthwhile to reiterate those characteristics that an adaptation model must meet and explain.

12.1.1 Action at a distance

Not withstanding that adaptation is spatially localized to the region of illumination (Chapter 10), it is clear that the effects of adaptation spread beyond the sites of photon absorption. In *Limulus* ventral photoreceptors, it has been directly shown that adaptation spreads somewhat beyond the region of illumination and that the spread cannot be accounted for by light scatter (Fein and Charlton, 1975*b*). Light adaptation of rods occurs at light intensities where only a few rhodopsin molecules are bleached per second. At such light intensities, the probability that the same disk absorbs the photons of both the adapting and test flashes is very low. Thus, the effects of adaptation are manifested not only by the disks that absorbed the photons but also by those that have not (Bastian and Fain, 1979). At the same time, the spread of adaptation in rods is such that it remains localized, that is, it does not spread more than about 10 μm from the site of photon absorption (see Chapter 10).

12.1.2 Increment–threshold curve

The way sensitivity varies with ambient light intensity is expressed by the increment–threshold curve. This relationship is illustrated in Figure 12.1 for invertebrate and vertebrate receptors. Such curves, which are plots of threshold versus intensity can be easily generated from data such as those in Figures 8.6 and 8.7, where the intensity–response curves were recorded for varying background intensities. More commonly, they are determined in a more direct manner, by superimposing, on a steady background light, a test flash whose intensity is varied to achieve a preselected criterion response. If the background is sufficiently dim, the cell does not light-adapt and the intensity of the test flash need not be increased. For the increment–threshold curve, which is a log–log plot, this absence of light adaptation with dim backgrounds is represented by the horizontal asymptote at the left of Figures 12.1*a* and *b*. With brighter backgrounds, log threshold rises linearly with the log of the light intensity. The slope of this linear region is typically less than one. The background light intensity corresponding to the intersection of the horizontal asymptote with the extrapolated linear region can be taken, for practical purposes, to characterize the light intensity at which adaptation begins to occur (see Figures 12.1*a* and *b*). It then represents the threshold of light adaptation. Chemical changes involved in adaptation would begin to occur at this light intensity and must be graded over the entire range of light intensities throughout which adaptation occurs. Rod photoreceptors are unlike others in that their adaptation range is limited (as was already indicated in Table 1.2 for humans). At a certain background intensity, even infinitely bright test flashes are unable to elicit a criterion response. This is shown in Figure 12.1*b* by the vertical asymptote.

12.1.3 Temporal requirements

In most photoreceptors, light adaptation occurs relatively rapidly, that is, within seconds. On the other hand, dark adaptation takes

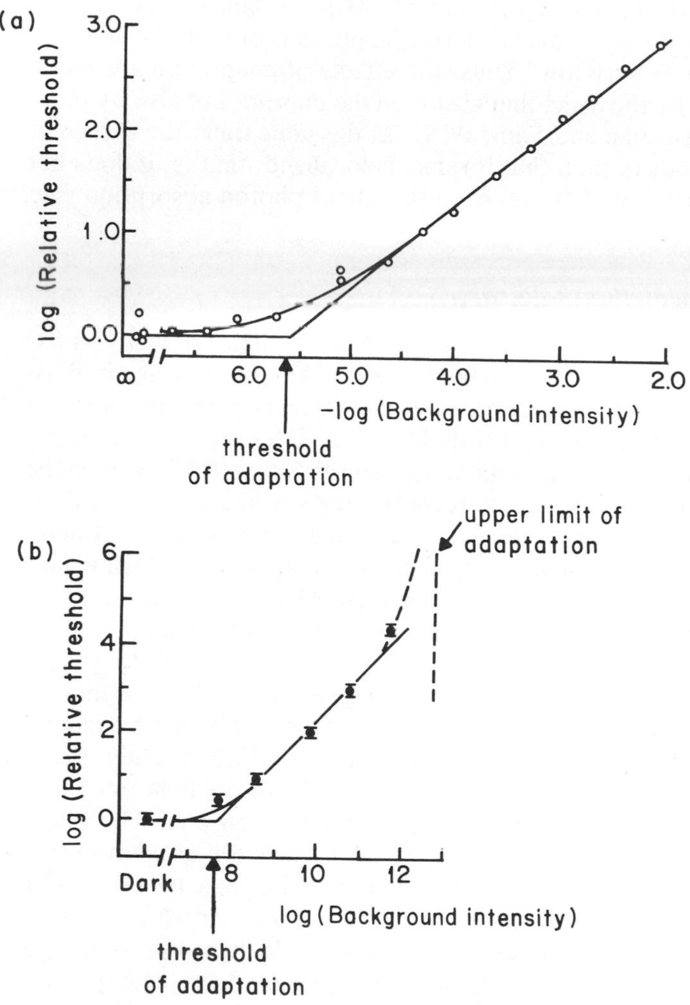

Figure 12.1. Increment–threshold curve for receptors. (*a*) *Limulus* ventral photoreceptor. (After Lisman and Strong, 1979) (*b*) Toad rods. (After Fain, 1976.)

minutes to an hour, depending on the light intensity and the particular photoreceptor (see Chapter 8). Thus it is difficult to put generalized temporal constraints on dark adaptation for all receptors.

12.2 Internal transmitter model for adaptation

As for excitation, a model incorporating an internal transmitter can satisfactorily explain the basic phenomenon of adaptation. Furthermore, all the preceding requirements can be satisfied whether light causes an increase or decrease in the concentration of the transmitter. If, for example, the absorption of light by rhodopsin would result in a rise in the concentration of a transmitter, then the localized spread of adaptation could be explained by the limited diffusion of the transmitter from the site of photon absorption. The time course of adaptation could be easily ascribed to specific release and uptake reactions. It is important to realize that the transmitter model for adaptation (or excitation for that matter) does not require that the transmitter be the sole arbiter of sensitivity. It could just as well be the initiator (trigger) of a series of complex multistep reactions.

At this point, it is appropriate to consider the implications of the constraints placed on the two transmitter models of excitation and adaptation. Could both be mediated by the same transmitter? If so, how could their concentration and their kinetics of release vary to fit the experimental observations? Because of the difference in time course between excitation and adaptation (for example, see Figure 8.8), it is clear that both processes cannot simply follow the concentration of one transmitter. Aside from the difference in time course, the other most noteworthy difference is that excitation is graded over only about 3 log units, whereas adaptation is usually graded over 6 or more log units. Numerous simple schemes can be provided to account for all of these observations. For example, let us say that the transmitter is released by light from some compartment. To satisfy the 3 log unit response range of excitation, it need only be true that the transmitter saturates some biochemical reaction; this might occur if there were a limited number of binding sites for the transmitter. Adaptation might simply be explained by light-induced changes in the ability of photoactivated rhodopsin to release transmitter. Submaximal release might occur either because rhodopsin was enzymatically modified so that it released less transmitter than in the dark-adapted cell or because the cell did not replenish the rhodopsin-sensitive compartment with a sufficient amount of transmitter. These changes in the efficiency of excitation would be graded over 6 or more log units. Such a scheme could account for excitation and adaptation with only one transmitter. Thus, the conservative idea of only one transmitter is viable. Surprisingly, the evidence that will be discussed in the next section, which indicates a role for Ca in adaptation of *Limulus* ventral photoreceptors, clearly rules out Ca as the excitatory transmitter in that cell. How well *Limulus* represents other receptors in this respect is not known. Because the ventral photoreceptor of *Limulus* is the receptor in which the molecular mechanisms of light adaptation have been most carefully investigated, it is appropriate that the rest of this chapter deal nearly exclusively with that cell.

12.3 Criteria to be met by a transmitter

The same requirements enumerated for excitation (see Chapter 11) hold for showing that a change in the concentration of some substance is involved in adaptation. As before, we shall consider each of Paton's criteria in turn.

12.4 Calcium as the internal transmitter

To discuss the role of calcium in adaptation when we have previously mentioned its possible role in excitation may seem paradoxical. The evidence for calcium's role in excitation comes primarily from vertebrate rods, the distal retina of the scallop, and the photosensitive neurons of *Aplysia*. Interestingly, all these photoreceptors hyperpolarize when illuminated, albeit their underlying permeability change is not necessarily to the same ion. On the other hand, the evidence for calcium's role in adaptation, which will be discussed later, comes primarily from *Limulus* ventral photoreceptors, which happen to depolarize when illuminated. Also, the evidence from ventral photoreceptors that suggests a role for calcium in adaptation seems to rule out the possibility that calcium is involved in excitation in that photoreceptor. Thus we have two separate sets of experimental evidence, one suggesting a role for calcium in excitation, the other in adaptation.

The suggestion that a light-induced rise in the intracellular cytoplasmic concentration of calcium is involved in the adaptation of *Limulus* ventral photoreceptors originated with Lisman and Brown (1972*a, b*). Their initial suggestion was based primarily on the observations that intracellular injection of Ca reduces the response to light, which is the essential effect of light adaptation.

Criterion 1. Presence of calcium in compartment from which it is released. There are basically only two compartments from which light could release calcium into the cytoplasm. Calcium either comes from outside (extracellular compartment) or from inside (intracellular compartment) the cell. Unfortunately, it is still not absolutely clear from which compartment the calcium that is released into the cytoplasm (see criterion 2) originates. On the one hand, it was suggested by Lisman and Brown that the source of calcium is an intracellular compartment (Brown and Blinks, 1974; Lisman, 1976), whereas Maaz and Stieve (1980) suggested that the extracellular space may be the compartment. Further work is needed to clarify this point. If the extracellular space turns out to be the source of calcium, then the normal 10-mM extracellular calcium concentration provides a nearly inexhaustible

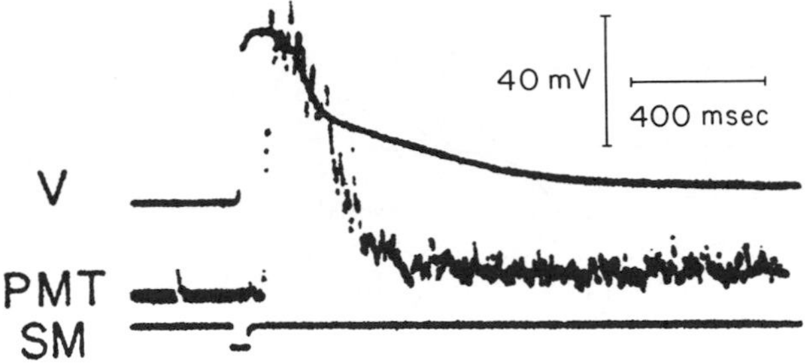

Figure 12.2. Light-induced rise in intracellular free calcium within *Limulus* ventral photoreceptor. Before the light stimulus, the cell was injected with aequorin, a water-soluble protein that luminesces in the presence of calcium. Its luminescence was detected with a photomultiplier tube, which collected the light emitted from the injected cell. The output signal from the photomultiplier (PMT) is shown on an arbitrary scale. The trace labeled V shows the simultaneously recorded membrane potential; the light stimulus is indicated by trace SM. (After Brown and Blinks, 1974.)

supply of calcium. If, however, the source of calcium is an intracellular compartment, then the identity of this compartment together with the amount of calcium it holds must be determined.

Criterion 2. Light effects on cytoplasmic calcium concentrations. If the hypothesis is correct, then an increase of the cytoplasmic calcium concentration should occur as a result of illumination. Brown and his colleagues (Brown and Blinks, 1974; Brown et al., 1977*b*) have successfully demonstrated such a rise using two completely independent methods (see Figure 12.2). However, two important questions still remain unanswered. First, do changes in intracellular calcium begin at the threshold of adaptation, and if so, are the changes graded over the entire range of adaptation? Second, is the rise of intracellular calcium as localized as light adaptation?

Criterion 3. Tests for identity of action. Light adaptation decreases not only the amplitude of the receptor response but also its latency (see Section 11.9). As Brown and Lisman (1975) showed, intracellular injection of calcium mimicked light in both of these respects (see Figure 12.3*a*). In addition, Fein and Charlton (1977*b*) showed that approximately the same quantitative relationship between sensitivity and latency exists whether desensitization is produced by light or by exogeneously injected calcium (see Figure 12.3*b*). Consideration of response latency is especially important because many processes can decrease

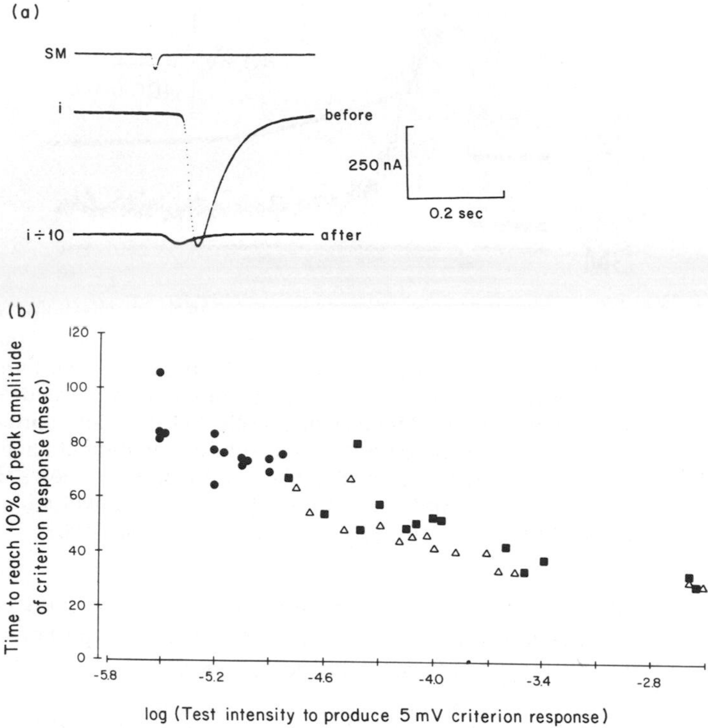

Figure 12.3. (*a*) Decrease in photoresponse amplitude and latency as a result of intracellular Ca injection. The light-induced current *i,* measured under voltage clamp, is shown before and after Ca injection. Response after injection is so small that it is shown here with a tenfold magnification. The occurrence of the test flash is shown by the stimulus monitor labeled SM. (After Brown and Lisman, 1975.) (*b*) Comparison of changes in sensitivity and latency produced by light adaptation and Ca injection. Controls (●) were obtained from dark-adapted receptors, which were not desensitized by light or calcium injection. The Ca injection (■) and light adaptation (△) data were obtained by desensitizing the receptor with the indicated procedure. (After Fein and Charlton, 1977*b*.)

sensitivity yet they may not also decrease latency. Anoxia, dinitrophenol, or carbon dioxide all desensitize *Limulus* photoreceptors, but they do not mimic light because they increase response latency (Lantz and Mauro, 1978).

Remember it was noted with regard to Figure 8.6 that the effect of adaptation is to shift the intensity–response curve along the intensity axis toward higher light intensities (also see Figure 8.7). If a rise in intracellular Ca is involved in adaptation, then one would predict that intracellular Ca injection would also cause the observed shifts for the intensity–response curves. Fein and Charlton (1977*b*) confirmed this prediction.

When ventral photoreceptors are repeatedly stimulated with light flashes near threshold, the individual responses exhibit considerable variability in their amplitude and latency. This response variability is believed to occur because of the variabilities in the amplitude, latency, and number of the quantum bumps, which summate to give the response (see Chapter 9). Fein and Charlton (1977*b*) found that the variabilities of response amplitude and of response latency decrease at threshold when the photoreceptor is desensitized by either light adaptation or calcium injection. Presumably, both light adaptation and calcium injection have similar effects on the underlying quantum bumps of the light response.

Ventral photoreceptors are sufficiently large so that small areas of the cell can be illuminated. Thus ventral photoreceptors are one of the few preparations where it was possible to demonstrate both localized excitation and adaptation (see Chapter 10). If the Ca hypothesis of Lisman and Brown is correct, then the injection of Ca into ventral photoreceptors could be predicted to lead to a localized desensitization of the cell. As shown in Figure 12.4, this prediction was confirmed.

An even more rigorous test of the hypothesis is a comparison of the kinetics of light and dark adaptation with that of the desensitization produced by calcium injection. Fein and Charlton (1978) found that the onset of desensitization during Ca injection was slower at the site of injection than the time course of light adaptation and the initial recovery from Ca injection was similarly slower than a comparable dark adaptation. The two time courses were only found to overlap during the final portions of the recovery from the adapting light or Ca injection. Though the discrepancy of these results may appear to be inconsistent with the Ca hypothesis, the results could be solely attributed to the fact that with exogenously injected calcium the release occurs from a point source much smaller than the diffuse area stimulated by the spot of light. Given the differences in geometry, the findings support and are consistent with the Ca hypothesis.

Criterion 4. Is a rise in intracellular calcium necessary for adaptation? The evidence just reviewed indicates that intracellular injection of Ca mimics many of the characteristics of light adaptation. However, none of those experiments address the question of whether a rise in intracellular Ca is a necessary condition for adaptation. Lisman and Brown (1975*b*) studied this question by injecting

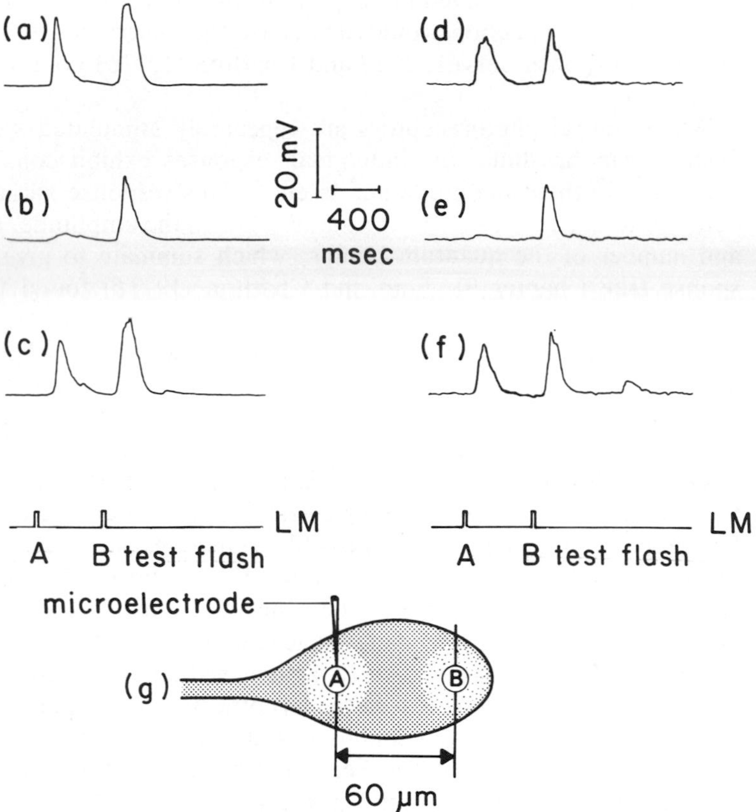

Figure 12.4. Localized desensitization produced by a local adapting light and by locally injected Ca. Part (*g*) is a schematized version of the photoreceptor, showing the two stimulus spots labeled A and B, with the intracellular Ca-containing electrode aligned with the spot at A. Two test flashes of constant intensity, one at A and one at B, were given in succession, as shown by the light monitor LM. Parts (*a*) and (*d*) show control responses elicited by the two spatially confined test flashes. Responses in (*b*) were recorded 3 sec after the occurrence of an adapting stimulus at A. The adapting stimulus greatly attenuated the response to the test flash at A, whereas the response to the flash at B was nearly unaffected. Responses in (*e*) were recorded after calcium injection at A. The injected calcium attenuated the response to the flash at A, leaving the response to the flash at B nearly unaffected. Parts (*c*) and (*f*) show that the cell completely recovered from the adapting stimulus and the calcium injection. (After Fein and Lisman, 1975.)

calcium buffers into ventral photoreceptors, with an aim to suppressing increases in intracellular calcium and thereby blocking adaptation. They found that injection of EGTA tended to prevent light-induced decreases in photoreceptor sensitivity. This result strongly supports the notion that changes in intracellular calcium are causally involved in adaptation.

Criterion 5. Presence of enzymes to regulate free calcium. As yet there is no convincing evidence to indicate the presence of the necessary enzymes or their location. Of course, the location of these enzymes will depend on the compartment from which calcium is released. There is still no consensus as to the identity of this compartment (see criterion 1).

In conclusion the preceding evidence clearly indicates that calcium plays an important role in adaptation of *Limulus* photoreceptors. Similar, but less extensive, studies indicate the same may be true for the honeybee drone (Bader et al., 1976). One obvious question that these findings raise is: what is the biochemical mechanism by which calcium modifies the sensitivity of the receptor? Unfortunately, at the present time, we know virtually nothing about the mechanism of this action.

12.5 Possible enzymatic reactions

As previously stated, adaptation (as excitation) involves complex biochemical reactions. Such reactions may play an integral role in the release of the transmitter and/or its eventual effect on the membrane permeability. Unfortunately, *Limulus* ventral photoreceptors are too few in number in any given animal to be a favorable preparation for biochemical studies. The identity of the reactions that may possibly be involved in adaptation comes from vertebrate rods, which provide adequate material for such biochemical studies. These possible reactions in vertebrates include the phosphorylation and dephosphorylation of rhodopsin.

Phosphorylation is the addition of phosphate to an organic compound, through the action of an enzyme termed a *kinase*. Rhodopsin from vertebrate rods is phosphorylated at sites exposed to the cytoplasm (Figure 4.3) by a reaction that is stimulated by light (Kühn and Dreyer, 1972; Bownds et al., 1972; Frank et al., 1973). The spectral sensitivity of rhodopsin phosphorylation in frog outer segments is similar to the absorption spectrum of rhodopsin. The enzyme (rhodopsin kinase) responsible for the reaction is a separate molecule from rhodopsin (Kühn et al., 1973; Weller et al., 1975; Miller and Paulsen, 1975). Light could initiate the phosphorylation reaction by either of two methods: either light causes an activation of the kinase or light causes a structural change in rhodopsin (the substrate), which exposes the phosphorylation site. The findings of Bownds et al. (1972) are consistent with the first mechanism, and the results of Kühn et al. (1973) and Frank and Bensinger (1974) seem to suggest the latter. The finding that the phosphorylation and dephosphorylation of rhodopsin occur in vivo (Kühn, 1974) strongly suggests that these reactions have some physiological significance. Because their rates are slow, they play a role more likely in adaptation than in excitation.

12.6 Summary

Very little experimental evidence is available on the biochemical reactions of adaptation. It has been suggested that a rise in the intracellular concentration of calcium is a factor involved in the adaptation of *Limulus* ventral photoreceptors and those of the honeybee drone. Several independent lines of evidence are consistent with this suggestion. However, very little detailed work has been performed to test the applicability of this suggestion to other photoreceptors.

REFERENCES

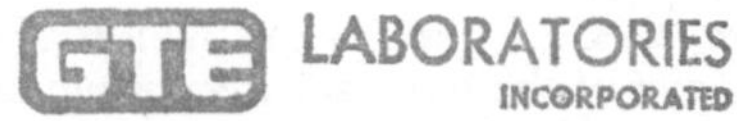

Adolph, A. (1964). Spontaneous slow potential fluctuations in the *Limulus* photoreceptor. *J. Gen. Physiol. 48*:297–322.

Adolph, A. (1968). Thermal and spectral sensitivities of discrete slow potentials in *Limulus* eye. *J. Gen. Physiol. 52*:584–99.

Akhtar, M., P. T. Blosse, and P. B. Dewhurst (1967). The active site of the visual protein, rhodopsin. *Chem. Comm.* 631–2.

Akimushkin, I. I. (1965). *Cephalopods of the Seas of the U.S.S.R.* Published for the Smithsonian Institution and the National Science Foundation, Washington, D.C., by Israel Program for Scientific Translation Ltd. (English translation, Golovonogie Mollyuski Morei SSSR, 1963).

Ali, M. A., ed. (1975). Retinomotor Responses in Vision in Fishes. In *New Approaches in Research,* Plenum, New York, pp. 313–55.

Ali, M. A. and M. Anctil (1976). *Retinas of Fishes: An Atlas.* Springer-Verlag, New York.

Andersen, M. C. and A. M. Brown (1979). Photoresponses of a sensitive extraretinal photoreceptor in *Aplysia. J. Physiol. 287*:267–82.

Andersen, M. C., A. M. Brown, and S. Yasui (1979). The role of diffusion in the photoresponse of an extraretinal photoreceptor of *Aplysia. J. Physiol. 287*:283–301.

Anderson, D. H. and S. K. Fisher (1975). Disc shedding in rodlike and conelike photoreceptors of tree squirrels. *Science 187*:953–5.

Arden, G. B. and J. C. Low (1978). Changes in pigeon cone photocurrent caused by reduction in extracellular calcium activity. *J. Physiol. 280*:55–76.

Arvanitaki, A. and N. Chalazonitis (1961). Excitatory and Inhibitory Processes Initiated by Light and Infra-red Radiations in Single Identifiable Nerve Cells (Giant Ganglion Cells of *Aplysia*). In *Nervous Inhibition,* E. Florey, ed. Pergamon Press, Elmsford, N.Y., pp. 194–231.

Azuma, K., M. Azuma, and W. Sickel (1977). Regeneration of rhodopsin in frog rod outer segments. *J. Physiol. 271*:747–59.

Bader, C. R., F. Baumann, and D. Bertrand (1976). Role of intracellular calcium and sodium in light adaptation in the retina of the honey bee drone (*Apis mellifera, L.*). *J. Gen. Physiol. 67*:475–91.

Bader, C. R., P. R. Macleish, and E. A. Schwartz (1979). A voltage-clamp study of the light response in solitary rods of the tiger salamander. *J. Physiol. 296*:1–26.

Ball, S., T. W. Goodwin, and R. A. Morton (1948). Studies on vitamin A.5:

The preparation of retinene$_1$–vitamin A aldehyde. *Biochem. J.* (London) *42*:516–23.
Barber, V. C., E. M. Evans, and M. F. Land (1967). The fine structure of the eye of the mollusc, *Pecten maximus*. *Z. Zellforsch. Mikrosk. Anat.* *76*:295–312.
Barlow, H. B. (1972). Dark and Light Adaptation. In *Handbook of Sensory Physiology,* vol. VII/4, D. Jameson and L. M. Hurvich, eds. Springer-Verlag, New York, pp. 1–28.
Barlow, R. B. and E. Kaplan (1971). *Limulus* lateral eye: properties of receptor units in the unexcised eye. *Science 174*:1027–9.
Barlow, R. B. and S. C. Chamberlain (1980). Light and a Circadian Clock Modulate Structure and Function in *Limulus* Photoreceptors. In *The Effects of Constant Light on Visual Processes*. T. P. Williams and B. N. Baker, eds. Plenum, New York.
Barlow, R. B., S. C. Chamberlain, and J. Z. Levinson (1980). *Limulus* brain modulates the structure and function of the lateral eye. *Science* *210*:1037–9.
Barr L. and M. Alpern (1963). Photosensitivity of the frog iris. *J. Gen. Physiol. 46*:1249–65.
Bastian, B. L. and G. L. Fain (1979). Light adaptation in toad rods: requirements for an internal messenger which is not calcium. *J. Physiol.* *297*:493–520.
Baumann, C. (1972). Kinetics of slow thermal reactions during the bleaching of rhodopsin in the perfused frog retina. *J. Physiol. 222*:643–63.
Baumann, C. (1976). The formation of metarhodopsin$_{380}$ in the retinal rods of the frog. *J. Physiol. 259*:357–66.
Baumann, C. and S. Bender (1973). Kinetics of rhodopsin bleaching in the isolated human retina. *J. Physiol. 235*:761–73.
Baur, P. S., Jr., A. M. Brown, T. D. Rogers, and M. E. Brown (1977). Lipochondria and the light response of *Aplysia* giant neurons. *J. Neurobiol. 8*:19–42.
Bayley, H., K.-S. Huang, R. Radhakrishnan, A. H. Ross, Y. Takagaki, and H. G. Khorana (1981). Site of attachment of retinal in bacteriorhodopsin. *Proc. Natl. Acad. Sci. U.S.A. 78*:2225–9.
Baylor, D. A. and R. Fettiplace (1975). Light path and photon capture in turtle photoreceptors. *J. Physiol. 248*:433–64.
Baylor, D. A. and M. G. F. Fuortes (1970). Electrical responses of single cones in the retina of the turtle. *J. Physiol. 207*:77–92.
Baylor, D. A. and A. L. Hodgkin (1973). Detection and resolution of visual stimuli by turtle photoreceptors. *J. Physiol. 234*:163–98.
Baylor, D. A. and A. L. Hodgkin (1974). Changes in time scale and sensitivity in turtle photoreceptors. *J. Physiol. 242*:729–58.
Baylor, D. A., Fuortes, M. G. F., and P. M. O'Bryan (1971). Receptive fields of single cones in the retina of the turtle. *J. Physiol. 214*:265–94.
Baylor, D. A., A. L. Hodgkin, and T. D. Lamb (1974). The electrical response of turtle cones to flashes and steps of light. *J. Physiol.* *242*:685–727.
Baylor, D. A., T. D. Lamb, and K. W. Yau (1979*a*). Responses of retinal rods to single photons. *J. Physiol. 288*:613–34.
Baylor, D. A., T. D. Lamb, and K. W. Yau (1979*b*). The membrane current of single rod outer segments. *J. Physiol. 228*:589–611.

Baylor, D. A., G. Mathews, and K. W. Yau (1980). Two components of electrical dark noise in toad retinal rod outer segments. *J. Physiol. 309*:591–621.

Bernard, G. D. (1979). Red absorbing visual pigment of butterflies. *Science 203*:1125–7.

Bertrand, D., M. G. F. Fuortes, and J. Pochobradsky (1978). Actions of EGTA and high calcium on the cones in the turtle retina. *J. Physiol. 275*:419–37.

Birge, R. R. (1981). Photophysics of light transduction in rhodopsin and bacteriorhodopsin. *Annu. Rev. Biophys. Bioeng. 10*:315–54.

Bitensky, M. W., R. E. Gorman, and W. H. Miller (1971). Adenyl cyclase as a link between photon capture and changes in membrane permeability of frog photoreceptors. *Proc. Natl. Acad. Sci. U.S.A. 68*:561–2.

Bito, L. Z. and D. G. Turansky (1975). Photoactivation of pupillary constriction in the isolated *in vitro* iris of a mammal (*Mesocricetus auratus*). *Comp. Biochem. Physiol. 50A*:407–13.

Blaurock, A. E. and M. H. F. Wilkins (1969). Structure of frog photoreceptor membranes. *Nature* (*London*) *223*:906–9.

Bogomolni, R. A., S. B. Hwang, Y. W. Tseng, G. I. King, and W. Stoeckenius (1977). Orientation of the bacteriorhodopsin transition dipole. *Biophys. J. 17*:98a (abstr.).

Bok, D. and M. O. Hall (1971). The role of the pigment epithelium in the etiology of inherited retinal dystrophy in the rat. *J. Cell. Biol. 49*:664–82.

Boll, F. (1876). Zur Anatomie und Physiologie der Retina. *Monatsber. dtsch. Akad. Wiss. Berlin 23*:783–7.

Boll, F. (1877). Zur Anatomie und Physiologie der Retina. *Arch. Anat. Physiol.* (*Physiol. Abt.*): 4–36. [An English translation appears in *Vision Res. 17*:1253–64 (1977)].

Borsellino, A. and M. G. F. Fuortes (1968). Responses to single photons in visual cells of *Limulus*. *J. Physiol. 196*:507–39.

Bowmaker, J. K. (1973). The photoproducts of retinal-based visual pigments *in situ:* a contrast between *Rana pipiens* and *Gekko gekko*. *Vision Res. 13*:1227–40.

Bowmaker, J. K. and H. J. A. Dartnall (1980). Visual pigments of rods and cones in a human retina. *J. Physiol. 298*:501–11.

Bownds, D. (1967). Site of attachment of retinal in rhodopsin. *Nature* (*London*) *216*:1178–81.

Bownds, D., J. Dawes, J. Miller, and M. Stahlman (1972). Phosphorylation of frog photoreceptor membranes induced by light. *Nature* (*London*), *New Biol. 237*:125–7.

Boynton, R. M. and D. N. Whitten (1970). Visual adaptation in monkey cones: recordings of late receptor potentials. *Science 177*:1423–6.

Bridges, C. D. B. (1967). Spectroscopic properties of porphyropsins. *Vision Res. 7*:349–69.

Bridges, C. D. B. (1971). The molar absorbance coefficient of rhodopsin. *Vision Res. 11*:841–8.

Bridges, C. D. B. (1972). The Rhodopsin–Porphyropsin Visual System. In *Photochemistry of Vision. Handbook of Sensory Physiology,* vol. VII/1, H. J. A. Dartnall, ed. Springer-Verlag, New York, pp. 417–80.

Bridges, C. D. B. (1976). Vitamin A and the role of the pigment epithelium

during bleaching and regeneration of rhodopsin in the frog eye. *Exp. Eye Res.* *22*:435–55.
Brin, K. P. and H. Ripps (1977). Rhodopsin photoproducts and rod sensitivity in the skate retina. *J. Gen. Physiol.* *69*:97–120.
Brindley, G. S. (1970). *Physiology of the Retina and Visual Pathway*. 2nd ed. Williams & Wilkins, Baltimore.
Brown, A. M. and H. M. Brown (1973). Light response of a giant *Aplysia* neuron. *J. Gen. Physiol.* *62*:239–54.
Brown, H. M., S. Hagiwara, H. Koike, and R. M. Meech (1970). Membrane properties of a barnacle photoreceptor examined by the voltage clamp technique. *J. Physiol.* *208*:385–413.
Brown, J. E. and J. R. Blinks (1974). Changes in intracellular free calcium concentration during illumination of invertebrate photoreceptors. Detection with aequorin. *J. Gen. Physiol.* *64*:643–65.
Brown, J. E. and J. A. Coles (1979). Saturation of the response to light in *Limulus* ventral photoreceptor. *J. Physiol.* *296*:373–92.
Brown, J. E. and J. E. Lisman (1972). An electrogenic sodium pump in *Limulus* ventral photoreceptor cells. *J. Gen. Physiol.* *59*:720–33.
Brown, J. E. and J. E. Lisman (1975). Intracellular Ca modulates sensitivity and time scale in *Limulus* ventral photoreceptors. *Nature* (*London*) *258*:252–4.
Brown, J. E. and M. I. Mote (1974). Ionic dependence of reversal voltage of the light response in *Limulus* ventral photoreceptors. *J. Gen. Physiol.* *63*:337–50.
Brown, J. E. and L. H. Pinto (1974). Ionic mechanisms for the photoreceptor potential of the retina of *Bufo marinus*. *J. Physiol.* *236*:575–91.
Brown, J. E., J. A. Coles, and L. H. Pinto (1977*a*). Effects of injections of calcium and EGTA into the outer segments of retinal rods of *Bufo marinus*. *J. Physiol.* *269*:707–22.
Brown, J. E., P. K. Brown, and L. H. Pinto (1977*b*). Detection of light-induced changes of intracellular ionized calcium concentration in *Limulus* ventral photoreceptors using Arsenazo III. *J. Physiol.* *267*:299–320.
Brown, J. E., H. H. Harary, and A. Waggoner (1979). Isopotentiality and an optical determination of series resistance in *Limulus* ventral photoreceptors. *J. Physiol.* *296*:357–72.
Brown, J. E. and G. Waloga (1981). Effects of cyclic nucleotides and calcium ions on *Bufo* rods. *Curr. Topics Membr. Transport* *15*:369–80.
Brown, K. T. and M. Murakami (1964). A new receptor potential of the monkey retina with no detectable latency. *Nature* (*London*) *201*:626–8.
Brown, P. K. (1972). Rhodopsin rotates in the visual receptor membrane. *Nature* (*London*), *New Biol.* *236*:35–8.
Brown, P. K. and G. Wald (1964). Visual pigments in single rods and cones of the human retina. *Science* *144*:45–52.
Burnside, B. (1976). Microtubules and actin filaments in teleost visual cone elongation and contraction. *J. Supramol. Struct.* *5*:257–75.
Burnside, B. and A. M. Laties (1979). Pigment Movement and Cellular Contractility in the Retinal Pigment Epithelium. In *The Retinal Pigment Epithelium,* K. M. Zinn and M. F. Marmor, eds. Harvard University Press, Cambridge, Mass., pp. 175–91.
Cafiso, D. S. and W. L. Hubbell (1980). Interfacial charge separation in photoreceptor membranes. *Photochem. Photobiol.* *32*:461–8.

Chabre, M. and A. Cavaggioni (1975). X-ray diffraction studies of retinal rods II. Light effect on the osmotic properties. *Biochim. Biophys. Acta 382*:336–43.

Chamberlain, S. C. and R. B. Barlow, Jr. (1979). Light and efferent activity control rhabdom turnover in *Limulus* photoreceptors. *Science 206*:361–3.

Clark, A. W. and D. Branton (1968). Fracture faces in frozen outer segments from the guinea pig retina. *Z. Zellforsch. Mikrosk. Anat. 91*:586–603.

Clark, A. W., R. Millecchia, and A. Mauro (1969). The ventral photoreceptor cells of *Limulus p*. The microanatomy. *J. Gen. Physiol. 54*:289–309.

Cohen, A. I. (1971). Electron microscope observations on form changes in photoreceptor outer segments and their saccules in response to osmotic stress. *J. Cell. Biol. 48*:547–65.

Cohen, A. I. (1972). Rods and Cones. In *Physiology of Photoreceptor Organs. Handbook of Sensory Physiology,* VII/2, M. G. F. Fuortes, ed. Springer-Verlag, New York, pp. 63–110.

Cohen, A. I. (1973). An ultrastructural analysis of the photoreceptors of the squid and their synaptic connections. I. Photoreceptive and nonsynaptic regions of the retina. *J. Comp. Neurol. 147*:351–78.

Coles, J. A. and J. E. Brown (1976). Effects of increased intracellular pH-buffering capacity on the light response of *Limulus* ventral photoreceptor. *Biochim. Biophys. Acta 436*:140–53.

Cone, R. A. (1964). Early receptor potential of the vertebrate retina. *Nature* (*London*) *204*:736–40.

Cone, R. A. (1967). Early receptor potential: photoreversible charge displacement in rhodopsin. *Science 155*:1128–31

Cone, R. A. (1972). Rotational diffusion of rhodopsin in the visual receptor membrane. *Nature* (*London*), *New Biol. 236*:39–43.

Cone, R. A. (1973). The Internal Transmitter Model for Visual Excitation: Some Quantitative Implications. In *Biochemistry and Physiology of Visual Pigments,* H. Langer, ed. Springer-Verlag, New York, pp. 275–82.

Cone, R. A. and W. H. Cobbs (1969). Rhodopsin cycle in the living eye of the rat. *Nature* (*London*) *221*:820–2.

Cone, R. A. and W. L. Pak (1971). The Early Receptor Potential. In *Principles of Receptor Physiology, Handbook of Sensory Physiology,* vol. I, W. R. Lowenstein, ed. Springer-Verlag, New York, pp. 345–65.

Cooper, A. (1979). Energy uptake in the first step of visual excitation. *Nature* (*London*) *282*:531–3.

Cornwall, M. C. and A. L. F. Gorman (1979). Contribution of calcium and potassium permeability changes to the off response of scallop hyperpolarizing photoreceptors. *J. Physiol. 291*:207–32.

Daemen, F. J. M., J. M. P. M. Borggreven, and S. L. Bonting (1970). Molar absorbance of cattle rhodopsin. *Nature* (*London*) *227*:1259–60.

Daemen, F. J. M., W. J. deGrip, and P. A. A. Jansen (1972). Biochemical aspects of the visual process XX. The molecular weight of rhodopsin. *Biochim. Biophys. Acta 271*:419–28.

Dartnall, H. J. A. (1952). Visual pigment 467, a photosensitive pigment present in tench retinae. *J. Physiol. 116*:257–89.

Dartnall, H. J. A. (1953). The interpretation of spectral sensitivity curves. *Br. Med. Bull. 9*:24–30.

Dartnall, H. J. A. (1968). The photosensitivities of visual pigments in the presence of hydroxylamine. *Vision Res. 8*:339–58.
Dartnall, H. J. A. (1972). Photosensitivity. In *Photochemistry of Vision, Handbook of Sensory Physiology,* vol. VII/1, H. J. A. Dartnall, ed. Springer-Verlag, New York, pp. 122–45.
Daw, N. W. and A. L. Pearlman (1974). Pigment migration and adaptation in the eye of the squid, *Loligo pealei. J. Gen. Physiol. 63*:22–36.
DeGrip, W. J., G. L. M. Van de Laar, F. J. M. Daemen, and S. L. Bonting (1973). Biochemical aspects of the visual process XXIII. Sulfhydryl groups and rhodopsin photolysis. *Biochim. Biophys. Acta 325*:315–22.
Detwiler, P. B. (1976). Multiple light-evoked conductance changes in the photoreceptors of *Hermissenda crassicornis. J. Physiol. 256*:691–708.
DeVoe, R. D. (1972). Dual sensitivities of cells in wolf spider eyes at ultraviolet and visible wavelengths of light. *J. Gen. Physiol. 59*:247–69.
Dodge, F. A., B. W. Knight, and J. Toyoda (1968). Voltage noise in *Limulus* visual cells. *Science 160*:88–90.
Donner, K. O. and T. Reuter (1968). Visual adaptation of the rhodopsin rods in the frog's retina. *J. Physiol. 199*:59–87.
Donner, K. O., S. Hemila, K. Hongell, and T. Reuter (1974). Long-lived photoproducts of porphyropsin in the retina of the crucian carp (*Carassius carassius*). *Vision Res. 14*:1359–70.
Dowling, J. E. (1960). The chemistry of visual adaptation in the rat. *Nature* (*London*) *188*:114–18.
Dowling, J. E. (1970). Organization of vertebrate retinas. *Invest. Ophthalmol. 9*:655–80.
Eakin, R. M. (1963). Lines of Evolution of Photoreceptors. In *General Physiology of Cell Specialization,* D. Mazia and A. Tyler, eds. McGraw-Hill, New York, pp. 393–425.
Eakin, R. M. (1972). Structure of Invertebrate Photoreceptors. In *Photochemistry of Vision, Handbook of Sensory Physiology,* vol. VII/1, H. J. A. Dartnall, ed. Springer-Verlag, New York, pp. 625–84.
Ebrey, T. G., and B. Honig (1975). Molecular aspects of photoreceptor function. *Quart. Rev. Biophys. 8*:129–84.
Ebrey, T. G., and B. Honig (1977). New wavelength dependent visual pigment nomograms. *Vision Res. 17*:147–51.
Edidin, M. (1974). Rotational and translocational diffusion in membranes. *Annu. Rev. Biophys. Bioeng. 3*:179–201.
Eisenbach, M. and S. R. Caplan (1979). The light-driven proton pump of *Halobacterium halobium*: mechanism and function. *Curr. Topics Membr. Transport 12*:165–248.
Engelman, D. E., R. Henderson, A. D. McLachlan, and B. A. Wallace (1980). Path of the polypeptide in bacteriorhodopsin. *Proc. Natl. Acad. Sci. U.S.A. 77*:2023–7.
Enoch, J. M. (1963). Optical properties of the retinal receptors. *J. Opt. Soc. Am. 53*:71–85.
Enoch, J. M. (1976). Vertebrate photoreceptor orientation. *Int. J. Quantum Chem.: Quantum Biology Symp. 3*:65–88.
Enoch, J. M. (1981). Retinal Receptor Orientation and Photoreceptor Optics. In *Vertebrate Photoreceptor Optics*, J. M. Enoch and F. L. Tobey, eds. Springer-Verlag, New York, pp. 127–68.
Enoch, J. M., D. G. Birch, and E. E. Birch (1979). Monocular light exclu-

sion for a period of days reduces directional sensitivity of the human retina. *Science 206*:705–7.

Ernst, W., C. M. Kemp, and H. A. White (1978). Studies on the effects of bleaching amphibian rod pigments *in situ*. II. The kinetics of the slow bleaching reactions in axolotl red rods. *Exp. Eye Res. 26*:337–350.

Exner, S. (1891). *Die Physiologie der facettieren Augen von Krebsen und Insekten* (*Physiology of Faceted Eyes of Crabs and Insects*). Deuticke, Vienna.

Fahrenbach, W. H. (1969). The morphology of the eyes of *Limulus* II. Ommatidia of the compound eye. *Z. Zellforsch. Mikrosk. Anat. 93*:451–83.

Fahrenbach, W. H. (1975). The visual system of the horseshoe crab, *Limulus polyphemus. Int. Rev. Cytol. 41*:285–349.

Fain, G. L. (1975). Quantum sensitivity of rods in the toad retina. *Science 187*:838–41.

Fain, G. L. (1976). Sensitivity of toad rods: dependence on wave-length and background illumination. *J. Physiol. 261*:71–101.

Fain, G. L. and J. E. Dowling (1973). Intracellular recordings from single rods and cones in the mudpuppy retina. *Science 180*:1178–81.

Falk, G. and P. Fatt (1966). Rapid hydrogen ion uptake of rod outer segments and rhodopsin solutions on illumination. *J. Physiol 183*:211–24.

Farber, D. B., D. W. Souza, D. G. Chase, and R. N. Lolley (1981). Cyclic nucleotides of cone-dominant retinas. Reduction of cyclic AMP levels by light and by cone degeneration. *Invest. Ophthalmol. Visual Sci. 20*:24–31.

Fatt, P. (1979). Decline of the calcium hypothesis of visual transduction. *Nature* (*London*) *280*:355–6.

Fein, A. and J. S. Charlton (1975*a*). Local membrane current in *Limulus* photoreceptors. *Nature* (*London*) *258*:250–2.

Fein, A. and J. S. Charlton (1975*b*). Local adaptation in the ventral photoreceptors of *Limulus. J. Gen. Physiol. 66*:823–36.

Fein, A. and J. S. Charlton (1977*a*). Enhancement and phototransduction in the ventral eye of *Limulus. J. Gen. Physiol. 69*: 553–69.

Fein, A. and J. S. Charlton (1977*b*). A quantitative comparison of the effects of intracellular calcium injection and light adaptation on the photoresponse of *Limulus* ventral photoreceptors. *J. Gen. Physiol. 70*: 591–600.

Fein, A. and J. S. Charlton (1978). A quantitative comparison of the time course of sensitivity changes produced by calcium injection and light adaptation in *Limulus* ventral photoreceptors. *Biophys. J. 22*:105–13.

Fein, A. and R. A. Cone (1973). *Limulus* rhodopsin: rapid return of transient intermediates to the thermally stable state. *Science 182*:495–7.

Fein, A. and D. W. Corson (1979). Both photons and fluoride ions excite *Limulus* ventral photoreceptors. *Science 204*:77–9.

Fein, A. and D. W. Corson (1981). Excitation of *Limulus* photoreceptors by vanadate and by an hydrolysis resistant analog of guanosine triphosphate. *Science 212*:555–7.

Fein, A. and R. D. DeVoe (1973). Adaptation in the ventral eye of *Limulus* is functionally independent of the photochemical cycle, membrane potential and membrane resistance. *J. Gen. Physiol. 61*:273–89.

Fein, A. and J. Lisman (1975). Localized desensitization of *Limulus* photoreceptors produced by light or intracellular calcium ion injection. *Science 187*:1094–6.

Findlay, J. B. C., M. Brett, and D. J. C. Pappin (1981). Primary structure of C-terminal functional sites in ovine rhodopsin. *Nature 293*:314–16.

Fineran, B. A. and J. A. C. Nicol (1976). Novel cones in the retina of the anchovy (*Anchoa*). *J. Ultrastruct. Res. 54*:296–303.

Fineran, B. A. and J. A. C. Nicol (1978). Studies on the photoreceptors of *Anchoa mitchilli* and *A. hepsetus* (Engraulidae) with particular reference to the cones. *Philos. Trans. R. Soc. London Ser. B. 283*:25–60.

Foster, M. C. (1980). Solution of the diffusion equation for membranes containing microvilli and lateral diffusion of rhodopsin and lipid analogs in squid photoreceptor membranes. *Fed. Proc. 39*:2067 (abstr.).

Frank, R. N. (1969). Photoproducts of rhodopsin bleaching in the isolated perfused frog retina. *Vision Res. 9*:1415–33.

Frank, R. N. (1971). Properties of neural adaptation in components of the frog electroretinogram. *Vision Res. 11*:1113–23.

Frank, R. N. and R. E. Bensinger (1974). Rhodopsin and light-sensitive kinase activity of retinal outer segments. *Exp. Eye Res. 18*: 271–80.

Frank, R. N. and J. E. Dowling (1968). Rhodopsin photoproducts: effects on electroretinogram sensitivity in isolated perfused rat retina. *Science 161*:487–9.

Frank, R. N., H. D. Cavanagh, and K. R. Kenyon (1973). Light-stimulated phosphorylation of bovine visual pigments by adenosine triphosphate. *J. Biol. Chem. 248*:596–609.

Frisch, K. von (1967). *The Dance Language and Orientation of Bees*. Harvard University Press, Cambridge, Mass. [English translation of *Tanzsprache und Orientierung der Bienen*. Springer-Verlag, New York, 1965.]

Fukuda, M. N., D. S. Papermaster, and P. A. Hargrave (1979). Rhodopsin carbohydrate: structure of small oligosaccharides attached at two sites near the NH_2 terminus. *J. Biol. Chem. 254*::8201–7.

Fung, B. K. K. and W. L. Hubbell (1978*a*). Organization of rhodopsin in photoreceptor membranes I. Proteolysis of bovine rhodopsin in native membranes and the distribution of sulfhydryl groups in the fragments. *Biochemistry 17*:4396–402.

Fung, B. K. K. and W. L. Hubbell (1978*b*). Organization of rhodopsin in photoreceptor membranes II. Transmembrane organization of bovine rhodopsin: evidence from proteolysis and lactoperoxidase-catalyzed iodination of native and reconstituted membranes. *Biochemistry 17*:4403–10.

Fung, B. K. K. and L. Stryer (1980). Photolyzed rhodopsin catalyzes the exchange of GTP for bound GDP in retinal rod outer segments. *Proc. Natl. Acad. Sci. U.S.A. 77*:2500–4.

Fung, B. K. K., J. B. Hurley, and L. Stryer (1981). Flow of information in the light triggered cyclic nucleotide cascade of vision. *Proc. Natl. Acad. Sci. U.S.A. 78*:152–6.

Fuortes, M. G. F. (1971). Generation of Responses in Receptor. In *Principles of Receptor Physiology*, W. R. Loewenstein, ed. Springer-Verlag, New York, pp. 243–68.

Fuortes, M. G. F. and A. L. Hodgkin (1964). Changes in time scale and sensitivity in the ommatidia of *Limulus*. *J. Physiol. 172*:239–63.

Fuortes, M. G. F. and P. M. O'Bryan (1972). Generator Potentials in Invertebrate Photoreceptors. In *Physiology of Photoreceptor Organs, Handbook of Sensory Physiology,* vol. II/2, M. G. F. Fuortes, ed. Springer-Verlag, New York, pp. 279–319.

Fuortes, M. G. F. and S. Yeandle (1964). Probability of occurrence of discrete potential waves in the eye of the *Limulus*. *J. Gen. Physiol.* *47*:443–63.

Futterman, S., J. C. Saari, and S. Blair (1977). Occurrence of a binding protein for 11-*cis* retinal in retina. *J. Biol. Chem.* *252*:3267–71.

Gogala, M. (1967). Die spektrale Empfindlichkeit der Doppel-augen von *Ascalaphus macaronius* Scop. (Neuroptera Ascalaphidae). *Z. Vergl. Physiol.* *57*:232–43.

Gold, G. H. and J. E. Dowling (1979). Photoreceptor coupling in retina of the toad, *Bufo marinus*. I. Anatomy. *J. Neurophysiol.* *42*:292–310.

Gold, G. H. and J. I. Korenbrot (1980). Light induced calcium release by intact retinal rods. *Proc. Natl. Acad. Sci. U.S.A.* *77*:5557–61.

Goldsmith, T. H. (1973). Photoreception and Vision. In *Comparative Physiology*, 3rd ed., C. L. Prosser ed. Saunders, Philadelphia, pp. 577–632.

Goldsmith, T. H. (1975). The Polarization Sensitivity–Dichroic Absorption Paradox in Arthropod Photoreceptors. In *Photoreceptor Optics*, A. W. Snyder and R. Menzel, eds. Springer-Verlag, New York, pp. 392–409.

Goldsmith, T. H. (1980). Hummingbirds see near ultraviolet light. *Science* *207*:786–8.

Goldsmith, T. H. and R. Wehner (1977). Restrictions on rotational and translational diffusion of pigment in the membranes of a rhabdomeric photoreceptor. *J. Gen. Physiol.* *70*:453–90.

Goldsmith, T. H., A. E. Dizon, and H. R. Fernandez (1968). Microspectrophotometry of photoreceptor organelles from eyes of the prawn *Palaemonetes*. *Science* *161*:468–70.

Goldstein, E. B. (1968). Visual pigments and the early receptor potential of the isolated frog retina. *Vision Res.* *8*: 953–64.

Goodeve, C. F., R. J. Lythgoe, and E. E. Schneider (1942). The photosensitivity of visual purple solutions and the scotopic sensitivity of the eye in the ultraviolet. *Proc. R. Soc. London, Ser. B* *130*:380–95.

Goridis, C., P. F. Urban, and P. Mandel (1977). The effect of flash illumination on the endogenous cyclic GMP content of isolated frog retinae. *Exp. Eye Res.* *24*:171–7.

Gorman, A. L. F. and J. S. McReynolds (1969). Hyperpolarizing and depolarizing receptor potentials in the scallop eye. *Science* *165*:309–10.

Gorman, A. L. F. and J. S. McReynolds (1974). Control of membrane K^+ permeability in the hyperpolarizing photoreceptor: similar effects of light and metabolic inhibitors. *Science* *185*:620–1.

Gouras, P. (1972). Light and Dark Adaptation. In *Physiology of Photoreceptor Organs, Handbook of Sensory Physiology,* vol. VII/2, M. G. F. Fuortes, ed. Springer-Verlag, New York, pp. 609–34.

Govardovskii, V. I. and A. L. Berman (1981). Light-induced changes of cyclic GMP content in frog retinal rod outer segments measured with rapid freezing and microdissection. *Biophys. Struct. Mech.* *7*:125–30.

Grabowski, S. R. and W. L. Pak (1975). Intracellular recordings of rod responses during dark-adaptation. *J. Physiol.* *247*:363–91.

Gray, E. G. and H. L. Pease (1971). On understanding the organization of the retinal receptor synapses. *Brain Res.* *35*:1–15.

Hagins, F. M. (1973). Purification and partial characterization of the protein component of squid rhodopsin. *J. Biol. Chem.* *248*:3298–304.

Hagins, W. A. (1955). The quantum efficiency of bleaching of rhodopsin *in situ*. *J. Physiol.* *129*:22 (abstr.).

Hagins, W. A. (1957). Rhodopsin in a Mammalian Retina. Ph.D. thesis, University of Cambridge.

Hagins, W. A. (1972). The visual process: excitatory mechanisms in the primary receptor cells. *Annu. Rev. Biophys. Bioeng.* *1*:131–58.

Hagins, W. A. and R. E. McGaughy (1967). Molecular and thermal origins of fast photoelectric effects of the squid retina. *Science* *157*:813–16.

Hagins, W. A. and S. Yoshikami (1974). A role for Ca^{++} in excitation of retinal rods and cones. *Exp. Eye Res.* *18*:299–305.

Hagins, W. A. and S. Yoshikami (1977). Intracellular Transmission of Visual Excitation in Photoreceptors: Electrical Effects of Chelating Agents Introduced into Rods by Vesicle Fusion. In *Vertebrate Photoreception,* H. B. Barlow and P. Fatt, eds. Academic Press, New York, pp. 97–139.

Hagins, W. A., H. V. Zonana, and R. G. Adams (1962). Local membrane current in the outer segments of squid photoreceptors. *Nature* (*London*) *194*:844–7.

Hagins, W. A., R. D. Penn, and S. Yoshikami (1970). Dark current and photocurrent in retinal rods. *Biophys. J.* *10*:380–412.

Hamasaki, D. I. and D. J. Eder (1977). Adaptive Radiations of the Pineal System. In *The Visual System in Vertebrates, Handbook of Sensory Physiology,* vol. VII/5, F. Crescitelli, ed. Springer-Verlag, New York, pp. 497–548.

Hamdorf, K. (1979). The Physiology of Invertebrate Visual Pigments. In *Comparative Physiology and Evolution of Vision in Invertebrates: Invertebrate Photoreceptors, Handbook of Sensory Physiology,* vol. VII/6A, H. Autrum, ed. Springer-Verlag, New York, pp. 145–224.

Hamdorf, K. and J. Schwemer (1975). Photoregeneration and the Adaptation Process in Insect Photoreceptors. In *Photoreceptor Optics,* A. W. Snyder and R. Menzel, eds. Springer-Verlag, New York, pp. 263–89.

Hamdorf, K., R. Paulsen, and J. Schwemer, (1973). Photoregeneration and Sensitivity Control of Photoreceptors of Invertebrates. In *Biochemistry and Physiology of Visual Pigments*. H. Langer, ed. Springer-Verlag, New York, pp. 155–66.

Hanani, M. and C. Shaw (1977). A potassium contribution to the response of the barnacle photoreceptor. *J. Physiol.* *270*:151–63.

Hargrave, P. A. and S.-L. Fong (1977). The amino- and carboxyl-terminal sequence of bovine rhodopsin. *J. Supramol. Struct.* *6*:559–70.

Hargrave, P. A., S. L. Fong, J. H. McDowell, M. T. Mas, and D. R. Curtis (1980). The partial primary structure of bovine rhodopsin and its topography in the retinal rod cell disc membrane. *Neurochem. Int.* *1*:231–44.

Harosi, F. I. (1975). Absorption spectra and linear dichroism of some amphibian photoreceptors. *J. Gen. Physiol.* *66*:357–82.

Harosi, F. I. (1976). Spectral relations of cone pigments in goldfish. *J. Gen. Physiol.* *68*:65–80.

Harosi, F. I. (1981). Microspectrophotometry and Optical Phenomena:

Birefringence, Dichroism and Anomalous Dispersion. In *Vertebrate Photoreceptor Optics, Springer Series in Optical Sciences,* vol. 23, J. M. Enoch and F. L. Tobey, eds., Springer-Verlag, New York, pp. 337–99.

Harosi, F. I. and E. F. MacNichol, Jr. (1974*a*). Dichroic microspectrophotometry: a computer assisted rapid wavelength-scanning photometer for measuring linear dichroism in single cells. *J. Opt. Soc. Am. 64*:908–18.

Harosi, F. I. and E. F. MacNichol, Jr. (1974*b*). Visual pigments of goldfish cones. Spectral properties and dichroism. *J. Gen. Physiol. 63*:279–304.

Harosi, F. I. and F. E. Malerba (1975). Plane polarized light in microspectrophotometry. *Vision Res. 15*:379–88.

Hartline, H. K. and F. Ratliff (1972). Inhibitory Interaction in the Retina of *Limulus*. In *Physiology of Photoreceptor Organs, Handbook of Sensory Physiology,* vol. VII/2, M. G. F. Fuortes, ed. Springer-Verlag, New York, pp. 381–447.

Hecht, S., S. Shlaer, and M. H. Pirenne (1942). Energy, quanta and vision. *J. Gen. Physiol. 25*:819–40.

Hecht, S., S. Shlaer, E. L. Smith, C. Haig, and J. C. Peskin (1948). The visual functions of the complete colorblind. *J. Gen. Physiol. 31*:459–72.

Heller, J. (1968). Structure of visual pigment. I. Purification, molecular weight and composition of bovine visual pigment 500. *Biochemistry 7*:2906–13.

Helverson, O. von and W. Edrich (1974). Der Polarizationsempfanger im Bienenauge: ein Ultraviolettrezeptor. *J. Comp. Physiol. 94*:33–47.

Henderson, R. and P. N. T. Unwin (1975). Three-dimensional model of purple membrane obtained by electron microscopy. *Nature (London) 257*:28–32.

Heyn, M. P., R. J. Cherry, and U. Muller (1977). Transient and linear dichroism on bacteriorhodopsin: determination of the orientation of the 568 nm all-trans retinal chromophore. *J. Mol. Biol. 117*:607–20.

Hillman, P., F. A. Dodge, S. Hochstein, B. W. Knight, and B. Minke (1973). Rapid dark recovery of the invertebrate early receptor potential. *J. Gen. Physiol. 62*:77–86.

Hodgkin, A. L. and P. M. O'Bryan (1977). Internal recording of the early receptor potential in turtle cones. *J. Physiol. 267*:737–66.

Hogan, M. J., Wood, I., and R. H. Steinberg (1974). Phagocytosis of pigment epithelium of human retinal cones. *Nature (London) 252*:305–7.

Hoglund, G. (1966). Pigment migration, light screening and receptor sensitivity in the compound eye of nocturnal lepidoptera. *Acta Physiol. Scand. 69*:282 (suppl.).

Honig, B. (1978). Light energy transduction in visual pigments and bacteriorhodopsin. *Annu. Rev. Phys. Chem. 29*:31–57.

Honig, B., U. Dinur, K. Nakanishi, V. Balogh-Nair, M. A. Gaminowicz, M. Arnaboldi, and M. G. Motto (1979). An external point-charge model for wavelength regulation in visual pigment. *J. Am. Chem. Soc. 101*:7084–6.

Horridge, G. A. and K. Mimura (1975). Fly photoreceptors I. Physical separation of two visual pigments in *Calliphora* retinula cells 1–6. *Proc. R. Soc. London, Ser. B 190*:211–24.

Horridge, G. A., C. Giddings, and G. Strange (1972). The superposition eye of skipper butterflies. *Proc. R. Soc. London, Ser. B 182*:457–95.

Hubbard, R. (1954). The molecular weight of rhodopsin and the nature of the rhodopsin digitonin complex. *J. Gen. Physiol. 37*:381–99.
Hubbard, R. (1958). The thermal stability of rhodopsin and opsin. *J. Gen. Physiol. 42*:259–80.
Hubbard, R. and A. Kropf (1958). The action of light on rhodopsin. *Proc. Natl. Acad. Sci. U.S.A. 44*:130–9.
Hubbard, R. and R. C. C. St. George (1958). The rhodopsin system of the squid. *J. Gen. Physiol. 41*:501–28.
Hubbard, R. and G. Wald (1952). *Cis–trans* isomers of vitamin A and retinene in the rhodopsin system. *J. Gen. Physiol. 36*:269–315.
Hubbard, R., D. Bownds, and T. Yoshizawa (1965). The chemistry of visual photoreception. *Cold Spr. Harbor Symp. Quant. Biol. 30*:301–15.
Huddleston, S. K. and T. P. Williams (1977). Physiological activity of isorhodopsin in rat rods. *Vision Res. 17*:711–14.
Hurvich, L. M. (1981). *Color Vision.* Sinauer, Sunderland.
Jacobs, S. F. (1978). Nonimaging Detectors. In *Handbook of Optics,* W. G. Driscoll and W. Vaughan, eds. McGraw-Hill, New York, pp. 4–1 to 4–69.
Jagger, W. S. (1979). Local stimulation and local adaptation of single isolated frog rod outer segments. *Vision Res. 19*:381–4.
Jan, L. Y. and Revel, J. P. (1974). Ultrastructural localization of rhodopsin in the vertebrate retina. *J. Cell. Biol. 62*:257–73.
Jones, C., J. Nolte, and J. E. Brown (1971). The anatomy of the median ocellus of *Limulus. Z. Zellforsch. Mikrosk. Anat. 118*:297–309.
Keefer, L. M. and R. A. Bradshaw (1977). Structural studies on *Halobacterium halobium* bacteriorhodopsin. *Fed. Proc. 36*:1799–804.
Keirns, J. J., N. Miki, M. W. Bitensky, and M. Keirns (1975). A link between rhodopsin and disc membrane cyclic nucleotide phosphodiesterase action spectrum and sensitivity to illumination. *Biochemistry 14*:2760–5.
Kilbride, P. and T. G. Ebrey (1979). Light-initiated changes of cyclic guanosine monophosphate levels in the frog retina measured with quick-freezing techniques. *J. Gen. Physiol. 74*:415–26.
Kirschfeld, K. (1965). Discrete and Graded Receptor Potentials in the Compound Eye of the Fly (*Musca*). In *The Functional Organization of the Compound Eye*, C. G. Bernhard ed. Pergamon Press, Elmsford, N.Y., pp. 291–307.
Kirschfeld, K., N. Franceschini, and B. Minke (1977). Evidence for a sensitizing pigment in fly photoreceptors. *Nature* (*London*) *269*:386–90.
Kleinschmidt, J. and J. E. Dowling (1975). Intracellular recordings from gecko photoreceptors during light and dark adaptation. *J. Gen. Physiol. 66*:617–48.
Koike, H., H. M. Brown, and S. Hagiwara (1971). Hyperpolarization of a barnacle photoreceptor membrane following illumination. *J. Gen. Physiol. 57*:723–37.
König, A. (1897). Die Abhangigkeit der Sehscharfe von Beleuchtungsintensitat. *Sitzungsber. K. Preuss. Akad. Wiss.* 559–75.
Korenbrot, J. I. and R. A. Cone (1972). Dark ionic flux and the effects of light in isolated rod outer segments. *J. Gen. Physiol. 60*:20–45.
Korenbrot, J. I., D. T. Brown, and R. A. Cone (1973). Membrane characteristics and osmotic behavior of isolated rod outer segments. *J. Cell Biol. 56*:389–98.

Kreithen, M. L. and T. Eisner (1978). Ultraviolet light detection by the homing pigeon. *Nature* (*London*) *272*:347–8.
Krohn, A. (1842). Nachtragliche Beobachtungen uber den Bau des Auges der Cephalopoden. *Verh. Kaiserlich Leopoldinisch–Carolinisch Dtsch. Acad. Naturforsch. XIX*(*2*):41–50.
Kropf, A. (1967). Intramolecular energy transfer in rhodopsin. *Vision Res. 7*:811–18.
Kropf, A. and R. Hubbard (1958). The mechanism of bleaching rhodopsin. *Ann. N.Y. Acad. Sci. 74*:266–80.
Kühn, H. (1974). Light-dependent phosphorylation of rhodopsin in living frogs. *Nature* (*London*) *250*: 588–90.
Kühn, H. and W. J. Dreyer (1972). Light dependent phosphorylation of rhodopsin by ATP. *FEBS Lett. 20*:1–6.
Kühn, H., J. H. Cook, and W. J. Dreyer (1973). Phosphorylation of rhodopsin in bovine photoreceptor membranes. A dark reaction after illumination. *Biochemistry 12*:2495–502.
Kühne, N. (1878). Zur Photochemie der Netzhaut. *Untersuch. Physiol. Inst. Univ. Heidelberg 1*:1–14.
Kunze, P. (1979). Apposition and Superposition Eyes. In *Comparative Physiology and Evolution of Vision in Invertebrates: Invertebrate Photoreceptors, Handbook of Sensory Physiology,* vol. VII/6A, H. Autrum, ed. Springer-Verlag, New York, pp. 441–502.
Labhart, T. (1980). Specialized photoreceptors at the dorsal rim of the honeybee's compound eye: polarizational and angular sensitivity. *J. Comp. Physiol. 141*:19–30.
Land, E. H. (1977). The retinex theory of color vision. *Sci. Am. 237*(*6*):108–28.
Land, M. F. (1979). The optical mechanism of the eye of *Limulus*. *Nature* (*London*) *280*:396–7.
Land, M. F. (1981). Optics and Vision in Invertebrates. In *Comparative Physiology and Evolution of Vision in Invertebrates: Invertebrate Visual Centers and Behavior I, Handbook of Sensory Physiology*, vol. VII/6B, H. Autrum, ed. Springer-Verlag, New York, pp. 471–592.
Langer, H. and B. Thorell (1966). Microspectrophotometry of single rhabdomeres in the insect eye. *Exp. Cell Res. 41*:673–7.
Lantz, R. C. and A. Mauro (1978). Alteration of sensitivity and time scale in invertebrate photoreceptors exposed to anoxia, dinitrophenol and carbon dioxide. *J. Gen. Physiol. 72*:219–31.
Larimer, J. L., D. L. Trevino, and E. A. Ashby (1966). A comparison of spectral sensitivities of caudal photoreceptors of epigeal and cavernicolous crayfish. *Comp. Biochem. Physiol. 19*:409–15.
Laties, A. M. (1969). Histological techniques for study of photoreceptor orientation. *Tissue Cell 1*:63–81.
Laties, A. M. and J. M. Enoch (1971). An analysis of retinal receptor orientation. I. Angular relationship of neighboring photoreceptors. *Invest. Ophthalmol. 10*:69–77.
LaVail, M. M. (1976*a*). Rod outer segment disc shedding in rat retina: relationship to cyclic lighting. *Science 194*:1071–4.
LaVail, M. M. (1976*b*). Survival of some photoreceptor cells in albino rats following long-term exposure to continuous light. *Invest. Ophthalmol. 15*:64–70.
LeGrand, Y. (1957). *Light, Colour and Vision.* Wiley, New York. [English

translation of *Optique Physiologique, Lumiere et Couleurs*, vol. II. Revue d'Optique, Paris, 1948.]

Levine, J. S. and E. F. MacNichol, Jr. (1979). Visual pigments in teleost fishes: effects of habitat, microhabitat, and behavior on visual system evolution. *Sensory Proc. 3*:95–131.

Levinson, J. Z. (1972). Interpretation of Generator Potentials. In *Physiology of Photoreceptor Organs, Handbook of Sensory Physiology*, vol. VII/2, M. G. F. Fuortes, ed. Springer-Verlag, New York, pp. 339–56.

Lewis, A. (1978*a*). The molecular mechanism of excitation in visual transduction and bacteriorhodopsin. *Proc. Natl. Acad. Sci. U.S.A. 75*:549–53.

Lewis, A. (1978*b*). The structure of the retinylidene chromophore in bathorhodopsin. *Biophys. J. 24*:249–54.

Lewis, M. S., L. C. Krieg, and W. D. Kirk (1974). The molecular weight and detergent binding of bovine rhodopsin. *Exp. Eye Res. 18*:29–40.

Liebman, P. A. (1962). In situ microspectrophotometric studies on the pigments of single retinal rods. *Biophys. J. 2*:161–78.

Liebman, P. A. (1975). Birefringence, Dichroism and Rod Outer Segment Structure. In *Photoreceptor Optics*, A. W. Snyder and R. Menzel, eds. Springer-Verlag, New York, pp. 199–214.

Liebman, P. A. (1978). Rod disk calcium movement and transduction: a poorly illuminated story. *Ann. N.Y. Acad. Sci. 307*:642–4.

Liebman, P. A. and G. Entine (1968). Visual pigments of frog and tadpole (*Rana pipiens*). *Vision Res. 8*:761–74.

Liebman, P. A. and G. Entine (1974). Lateral diffusion of visual pigment in photoreceptor disk membranes. *Science 185*:457–9.

Liebman, P. A. and A. M. Granda (1975). Super dense carotenoid spectra resolved in single cone oil droplets. *Nature* (*London*) *253*:370–2.

Liebman, P. A. and E. N. Pugh (1980). ATP mediates rapid reversal of cyclic GMP phosphodiesterase activation in visual receptor membranes. *Nature* (*London*) *287*:734–6.

Liebman, P. A., S. Carroll, and A. Laties (1969). Spectral sensitivity of retinal screening pigment migration in the frog. *Vision Res. 9*:377–84.

Lillywhite, P. G. (1977). Single photon signals and transduction in an insect eye. *J. Comp. Physiol. 122*:189–200.

Lipton, S. A., S. E. Ostroy, and J. E. Dowling (1977*a*). Electrical and adaptive properties of rod photoreceptors in *Bufo marinus* I. Effects of altered extracellular Ca^{++} levels. *J. Gen. Physiol. 70*:747–70.

Lipton, S. A., H. Rasmussen, and J. E. Dowling (1977*b*). Electrical and adaptive properties of rod photoreceptor in *Bufo marinus* II. Effects of cyclic nucleotide and prostaglandins. *J. Gen. Physiol. 70*:771–91.

Lisman, J. E. (1976). Effects of removing extracellular Ca^{++} on excitation and adaptation in *Limulus* ventral photoreceptors. *Biophys. J. 16*:1331–5.

Lisman, J. E. and H. Bering (1977). Electrophysiological measurement of the number of rhodopsin molecules in single *Limulus* photoreceptors. *J. Gen. Physiol. 70*:621–33.

Lisman, J. E. and J. E. Brown (1972*a*). The Effects of Intracellular Ca^{++} on the Light Response and on Light Adaptation in *Limulus* Ventral Photoreceptors. In *The Visual System: Neurophysiology, Biophysics and Their Clinical Applications*, G. B. Arden, ed. Plenum, New York, pp. 23–33.

Lisman, J. E. and J. E. Brown (1972*b*). The effects of intracellular iontophoretic injection of calcium and sodium ions on the light response of *Limulus* ventral photoreceptors. *J. Gen. Physiol. 59*:701–19.
Lisman, J. E. and J. E. Brown (1975*a*). Light-induced changes of sensitivity in *Limulus* ventral photoreceptors. *J. Gen. Physiol. 66*:473–88.
Lisman, J. E. and J. E. Brown (1975*b*). Effects of intracellular injection of calcium buffers in *Limulus* ventral photoreceptors. *J. Gen. Physiol. 66*:489–506.
Lisman, J. E. and Y. Sheline (1976). Analysis of the rhodopsin cycle in *Limulus* ventral photoreceptors using the early receptor potential. *J. Gen. Physiol. 68*:487–501.
Lisman, J. E. and J. A. Strong (1979). The initiation of excitation and light adaptation in *Limulus* ventral photoreceptors. *J. Gen. Physiol. 73*:219–43.
Loew, E. R. and H. J. A. Dartnall (1976). Vitamin A_1/A_2-based visual pigment mixtures in cones of the rudd. *Vision Res. 16*:891–6.
Maaz, G. and H. Stieve (1980). The correlation of the receptor potential with the light induced transient increase in intracellular calcium-concentration measured by absorption change of Arsenazo III injected into *Limulus* ventral nerve photoreceptor cell. *Biophys. Struct. Mech. 6*:191–208.
Marks, W. B., W. H. Dobelle, and E. F. MacNichol, Jr. (1964). Visual pigments of single primate cones. *Science 143*:1181–3.
Matthews, R. G., R. Hubbard, P. K. Brown, and G. Wald (1963). Tautomeric forms of metarhodopsin. *J. Gen. Physiol. 47*:215–40.
McFarland, W. N. and F. W. Munz (1975). The Visible Spectrum During Twilight and Its Implications to Vision. In *Light as an Ecological Factor*, vol. II, G. C. Evans, R. Bainbridge, and O. Rackham, eds., Blackwell Sci. Publ., Oxford, pp. 249–70.
McNaughton, P. A., K. W. Yau, and T. D. Lamb (1980). Spread of activation and desensitization in rod outer segments. *Nature (London) 283*:85–7.
McReynolds, J. S. and A. L. F. Gorman (1970*a*). Photoreceptor potentials of opposite polarity in the eye of the scallop, *Pecten irradians*. *J. Gen. Physiol. 56*:376–91.
McReynolds, J. S. and A. L. F. Gorman (1970*b*). Membrane conductances and spectral sensitivities of *Pecten* photoreceptors. *J. Gen. Physiol. 56*:392–406.
McReynolds, J. S. and A. L. F. Gorman (1974). Ionic basis of hyperpolarizing receptor potential in scallop eye: increase in permeability to potassium ions. *Science 183*:658–9.
Menzel, R. (1975). Polarization Sensitivity in Insect Eyes with Fused Rhabdoms. In *Photoreceptor Optics*, A. W. Snyder and R. Menzel, eds. Springer-Verlag, New York, pp. 372–7.
Menzel, R. and M. Blakers (1976). Colour receptors in the bee eye – morphology and spectral sensitivity. *J. Comp. Physiol. 108*:11–33.
Miki, N., J. M. Baraban, J. J. Keirns, J. J. Boyce, and M. W. Bitensky (1975). Purification and properties of the light-activated cyclic nucleotide phosphodiesterase of rod outer segments. *J. Biol. Chem. 250*:6320–7.
Millecchia, R. and A. Mauro (1969). The ventral photoreceptor cells of *Limulus* III. A voltage-clamp study. *J. Gen. Physiol. 54*:331–51.

Miller, J. A. and R. Paulsen (1975). Phosphorylation and dephosphorylation of frog rod outer segment membranes as part of the visual process. *J. Biol. Chem. 250*:4427–32.

Miller, W. H. and G. D. Nicol (1979). Evidence that cyclic GMP regulates membrane potential in rod photoreceptors. *Nature* (*London*) *280*:64–6.

Minke, B., S. Hochstein, and P. Hillman (1973). Early receptor potential evidence for the existence of two thermally stable states in the barnacle visual pigment. *J. Gen. Physiol. 62*:87–104.

Müller, H. (1851). Zur Histologie der Retina. *Z. Wiss. Zool. 3*:234–7.

Munk, O. (1966). Ocular anatomy of some deep sea teleosts. Dana Report No. 70, pp. 1–71.

Munz, F. W. and S. A. Schwanzara (1967). A nomogram of retinene$_2$-based visual pigments. *Vision Res. 7*:111–20.

Murakami, M. and W. L. Pak (1970). Intracellularly recorded early receptor potential of the vertebrate photoreceptors. *Vision Res. 10*:965–75.

Naka, K. I. and W. A. H. Rushton (1966). S-potentials from colour units in the retina of fish (Cyprinidae). *J. Physiol. 185*:536–55.

Nilsson, S. E. G. (1964). An electron microscopic classification of the retinal receptors of the leopard frog (*Rana pipiens*). *J. Ultrastruct. Res. 10*:390–416.

Oseroff, A. R. and R. H. Callender (1974). Resonance Raman spectroscopy of rhodopsin in retinal disc membranes. *Biochemistry 13*:4243–8.

Østerberg, G. (1935). Topography of the layer of rods and cones in the human retina. *Acta Ophthalmol. Kbh.* Suppl. 6.

Ovchinnikov, Y. A., N. G. Abdulaev, M. Y. Feigina, A. V. Kiselev, and N. A. Lobanov (1979). The structural basis of the functioning of bacteriorhodopsin: an overview. *FEBS Lett. 100*:219–24.

Owen, J. D. and H. M. Brown (1980). Intracellular changes of H^+ and Ca^{++} activities in *Aplysia* giant neurons as measured with ion selective microelectrodes. *Comp. Biochem. Physiol. 66*:197–201.

Pak, W. L. and R. A. Cone (1964). Isolation and identification of the initial peak of the early receptor potential. *Nature* (*London*) *204*:836–8.

Paton, W. D. M. (1958). Central and synaptic transmission in the nervous system (pharmacological aspects). *Annu. Rev. Physiol. 20*:431–70.

Penn, R. D. and W. A. Hagins (1972). Kinetics of the photocurrent of retinal rods. *Biophys. J. 12*:1073–94.

Pepose, J. S. and J. E. Lisman (1978). Voltage sensitive potassium channels in *Limulus* ventral photoreceptors. *J. Gen. Physiol. 71*:101–20.

Pepperberg, D. R., M. Lurie, P. K. Brown, and J. E. Dowling (1976). Visual adaptation: effects of externally applied retinal on the light-adapted isolated skate retina. *Science 191*:394–6.

Pepperberg, D. R., P. K. Brown, M. Lurie, and J. E. Dowling (1978). Visual pigment and photoreceptor sensitivity in the isolated skate retina. *J. Gen. Physiol. 71*:369–96.

Peters, K., M. L. Applebury, and P. M. Rentzepis (1977). Primary photochemical event in vision: proton translocation. *Proc. Natl. Acad. Sci. U.S.A. 74*:3119–23.

Petersen, D. C. and R. A. Cone (1975). The electric dipole moment of rhodopsin solubilized in Triton X-100. *Biophys. J. 15*:1181–200.

Pinto, L. H. and S. E. Ostroy (1978). Ionizable groups and conductance of the rod photoreceptor membrane. *J. Gen. Physiol. 71*:329–45.

Pirenne, M. H. (1962). Absolute Thresholds and Quantum Effects. In *The Eye,* J. Davson, ed. Academic Press, New York, pp. 123–40.
Pirenne, M. H., F. H. C. Marriott, and E. F. O'Doherty (1957). Individual differences in night-vision efficiency. *Med. Res. Coun. (GB) Spec. Rep. Ser. 294.*
Plantner, J. J. and E. L. Kean (1976). Carbohydrate composition of bovine rhodopsin. *J. Biol. Chem. 251*:1548–52.
Pober, J. S. and M. W. Bitensky (1979). Light-regulated enzymes of vertebrate retinal rods. *Adv. Cyclic Nucleotide Res. 11*:266–301.
Polans, A. S., S. Kawamura, and M. D. Bownds (1981). Influence of calcium on guanosine 3′, 5′-cyclic monophosphate levels in frog rod outer segments. *J. Gen. Physiol. 77*:41–8.
Poo, M. M. and R. A. Cone (1974). Lateral diffusion of rhodopsin in the photoreceptor membrane. *Nature (London) 247*:438–41.
Pratt, D. C. (1968). Photoreactions of isorhodopsin at low temperatures. *Photochem. Photobiol. 7*:319–24.
Reuter, T. (1976). Photoregeneration of rhodopsin and isorhodopsin from metarhodopsin III in the frog retina. *Vision Res. 16*:909–17.
Reuter, T. E., R. H. White, and G. Wald (1971). Rhodopsin and porphyropsin fields in the adult bullfrog retina. *J. Gen. Physiol. 58*:351–71.
Reyer, R. W. (1977). The Amphibian Eye: Development and Regeneration. In *The Visual System in Vertebrates, Handbook of Sensory Physiology,* vol. VII/5, F. Crescitelli, ed. Springer-Verlag, New York, pp. 309–90.
Robinson, W. E. and W. A. Hagins (1979). GTP hydrolysis in intact rod outer segments and the transmitter cycle in visual excitation. *Nature (London) 280*:398–400.
Robinson, W. E. and W. A. Hagins (1980). Bound and free nucleotides in rod outer segments. *Fed. Proc. 39*:2067 (abstr.).
Robinson, W. E., A. Gordon-Walker, and D. Bownds (1972). Molecular weight of frog rhodopsin. *Nature (London) New Biol. 235*:112–14.
Rodieck, R. W. (1973). *The Vertebrate Retina: Principles of Structure and Function.* Freeman, San Francisco.
Röhlich, P. (1976). Photoreceptor membrane carbohydrate on the intradiscal surface of retinal rod disks. *Nature (London) 263*:789–91.
Rossel, S. (1979). Regional differences in photoreceptor performance in the eye of the praying mantis. *J. Comp. Physiol. 131*:95–112.
Rothschild, K. J., J. R. Andrew, W. J. DeGrip, and H. E. Stanley (1976). Opsin structure probed by Raman spectroscopy of photoreceptor membranes. *Science 191*:1176–8.
Rüppel, H. and W. A. Hagins (1973). Spatial Origin of the Fast Photovoltage in Retinal Rods. In *Biochemistry and Physiology of Visual Pigments*, H. Langer, ed. Springer-Verlag, New York, pp. 257–61.
Rushton, W. A. H. (1957). Physical measurements of cone pigment in the living human eye. *Nature (London) 179*:571–3.
Rushton, W. A. H. (1961). Rhodopsin measurement and dark-adaptation in a subject deficient in cone vision. *J. Physiol. 156*:193–205.
Rushton, W. A. H. (1963). A cone pigment in the protanope. *J. Physiol. (London) 168*:345–59.
Rushton, W. A. H. (1965). A foveal pigment in the deuteranope. *J. Physiol. (London) 176*:24–37.
Rushton, W. A. H. (1972). Visual Pigments in Man. In *Photochemistry of*

Vision, Handbook of Sensory Physiology, H. J. A. Dartnall, ed. Springer-Verlag, New York, pp. 364–94.

Rushton, W. A. H., F. W. Campbell, W. A. Hagins, and G. S. Brindley (1955). The bleaching and regeneration of rhodopsin in the living eye of the albino rabbit and of man. *Optica Acta 1*:183–90.

Saari, J. C. and S. Futterman (1976). Retinal-binding protein in bovine retina: isolation and partial characterization. *Exp. Eye Res. 22*:425–33.

Schmidt, J. A. and D. B. Farber (1980). Light-induced changes in *c*AMP levels in *Limulus* photoreceptors. *Biochem. Biophys. Res. Comm. 94*:438–42.

Schneider, L., M. Gogala, K. Draslar, H. Langer, and P. Schlecht (1978). Feinstruktur und Schirmpigment–Eigenschaften der Ommatidien des Doppelauges von Ascalaphus (Insecta, Neuroptera). *Cytobiologie 16*:274–307.

Scholes, J. (1965). Discontinuity of the excitation process in locust visual cells. *Cold Spr. Harbor Symp. Quant. Biol. 30*:517–27.

Scholes, J. (1969). The electrical responses of the retinal receptors and the lamina in the visual system of the fly *Musca. Kybernetik 6*:149–62.

Schultze, M. (1866). Zur Anatomie und Physiologie der Retina. *Arch. Mikrosk. Anat. 2*:175–86.

Schwartz, S., L. B. Lerch, and E. A. Dratz (1977). The sulfhydryl-disulfide content of rhodopsin. *J. Gen. Physiol. 70*:169 (abstr.).

Schwemer, J. (1969). Der Sehfarbstoff von *Eledone moschata* und seine Umsetzung in der lebenden Netzhaut. *Z. Vergl. Physiol. 62*:121–52.

Schwemer, J. and R. Paulsen (1973). Three visual pigments in *Deilephila elpenor* (Lepidoptera Sphingidae), *J. Comp. Physiol. 86*:215–29.

Schwemer, J., M. Gogola, and K. Hamdorf (1971). Der UV-Sehfarbstoff der Insekten: Photochemie in vitro und in vivo. *Z. Vergl. Physiol. 75*:174–88.

Seldin, E. B., R. H. White, and P. K. Brown (1972). Spectral sensitivity of larval mosquito ocelli. *J. Gen. Physiol. 59*:415–20.

Seliger, H. H. (1977). Environmental Photobiology. In *The Science of Photobiology*, K. C. Smith, ed. Plenum, New York, pp. 143–73.

Seliger, H. H. and W. D. McElroy (1965). *Light: Physical and Biological Action*. Academic Press, New York.

Shaw, S. R. (1969). Sense-cell structure and interspecies comparisons of polarized-light absorption in arthropod compound eyes. *Vision Res. 9*:1031–40.

Sherk, T. E. (1978). Development of the compound eyes of dragonflies (Odonata) III. Adult compound eyes. *J. Exp. Zool. 203*:61–80.

Shichi, H. (1971). Circular dichroism of bovine rhodopsin. *Photochem. Photobiol. 13*:499–502.

Shichi, H. and E. Shelton (1974). Assessment of physiological integrity of sonicated retinal rod membranes. *J. Supramol. Struct. 2*:7–16.

Shichi, H., M. S. Lewis, F. Irreverre, and A. L. Stone (1969). Biochemistry of visual pigment. I. Purification and properties of bovine rhodopsin. *J. Biol. Chem. 244*:529–536.

Shinozawa, T., I. Sen, G. Wheeler, and M. Bitensky (1979). Predictive value of the analogy between hormone-sensitive adenylate cyclase and light-sensitive photoreceptor cyclic GMP phosphodiesterase: a specific role for a light-sensitive GTPase as a component in the activation sequence. *J. Supramol. Struct. 10*:185–90.

Shinozawa, T., S. Uchida, E. Martin, D. Cafiso, W. Hubbell, and M. Bitensky (1980). Additional components required for activity and reconstitution of light-activated vertebrate photoreceptor GTPase. *Proc. Natl. Acad. Sci. U.S.A. 77*:1408–11.

Shlaer, R. (1972). An eagle's eye: quality of the retinal image. *Science 176*:920–2.

Shlaer, S. (1937). The relation between visual acuity and illumination. *J. Gen. Physiol. 21*:165–88.

Sickel, W. (1965). Respiratory and electrical responses to light stimulation in the retina of the frog. *Science 148*:648–51.

Smith, C. A. and F. S. Sjöstrand (1961). A synaptic structure in the hair cells of the guinea pig cochlea. *J. Ultrastruct. Res. 5*:184–92.

Smith, H. G., R. S. Fager, and B. J. Litman (1977). Light-activated calcium release from sonicated bovine retinal rod outer segment disks. *Biochemistry 16*:1399–405.

Smith, T. G. and F. Baumann (1969). The Functional Organization within the Ommatidium of the Lateral Eye of *Limulus*. In *Mechanisms of Synaptic Transmission, Progress in Brain Research*, vol. 31, K. Akert and P. G. Waser, eds. Elsevier, North-Holland, New York. pp. 313–49.

Snyder, A. W. (1979). The Physics of Vision in Compound Eyes. In *Comparative Physiology and Evolution of Vision in Invertebrates: Invertebrate Photoreceptors, Handbook of Sensory Physiology*, vol. VII/6A, H. Autrum, ed. Springer-Verlag, New York, pp. 225–314.

Snyder, A. W., R. Menzel, and S. B. Laughlin (1973). Structure and function of the fused rhabdom. *J. Comp. Physiol. 87*:99–135.

Srebro, R. and M. Behbehani (1972). The thermal origin of spontaneous activity in the *Limulus* photoreceptor. *J. Physiol. 224*:349–61.

Stell, W. K. and F. I. Harosi (1976). Cone structure and visual pigment content in the retina of the goldfish. *Vision Res. 16*:647–57.

Stubbs, G. W., H. G. Smith, Jr., and B. J. Litman (1976). Alkyl glucosides as effective solubilizing agents for bovine rhodopsin. A comparison with several commonly used detergents. *Biochim. Biophys. Acta 426*:46–56.

Szuts, E. Z. (1975). Calcium content of the frog rod outer segment: effects of light and hypotonic lysis. Ph.D. thesis, Johns Hopkins University.

Szuts, E. Z. (1980). Calcium flux across disk membranes: studies with intact rod photoreceptors and purified disks. *J. Gen. Physiol. 76*:253–86.

Szuts, E. Z. and R. A. Cone (1977). Calcium content of frog rod outer segments and discs. *Biochim. Biophys. Acta 468*:194–208.

Tomita, T. (1970). Electrical activity of vertebrate photoreceptors. *Quart. Rev. Biophys. 3*:179–222.

Trujillo-Cenoz, O. (1965). Some aspects of the structural organization of the arthropod eye. *Cold Spr. Harbor Symp. Quant. Biol. 30*:371–82.

Wald, G. (1933). Vitamin A in the retina. *Nature* (*London*) *132*:316–17.

Wald, G. (1935). Carotenoids and the visual cycle. *J. Gen. Physiol. 19*:351–71.

Wald, G. (1945). Human vision and the spectrum. *Science 101*:653–8.

Wald, G. (1953). The biochemistry of vision. *Annu. Rev. Biochem. 22*:497–526.

Wald, G. (1968). Molecular basis of visual excitation. *Science 162*:230–9.

Wald, G. and S. Rayport (1977). Vision in annelid worms. *Science 196*:1434–9.

Wald, G., P. K. Brown, and P. H. Smith (1953). Cyanopsin, a new pigment of cone vision. *Science 118*:505–8.
Wald, G., P. K. Brown, and P. H. Smith (1955). Iodopsin. *J. Gen. Physiol. 38*:623–81.
Wald, G., P. K. Brown, and I. R. Gibbons (1963). The problem of visual excitation. *J. Opt. Soc. Am. 53*:20–35.
Walls, G. L. (1942). *The Vertebrate Eye and Its Adaptive Radiation* Cranbook Press, Michigan.
Waloga, G. and M. W. Bitensky (1981). Receptor potentials generated in the presence of non-hydrolysable analogs of cyclic GMP. *Invest. Ophthalmol. Visual Sci. 20*:223(ARVO abstr.).
Walther, J. B. (1965). Single Cell Responses from the Primitive Eyes of an Annelid. In *The Functional Organization of the Compound Eye*, C. G. Bernhard, ed. Pergamon Press, Elmsford, N.Y., pp. 329–36.
Wang, J. K., J. H. McDowell, and P. A. Hargrave (1980). Site of attachment of 11-*cis*-retinal in bovine rhodopsin. *Biochemistry 19*:5111–17.
Waterman, T. H. (1981). Polarization Sensitivity. In *Comparative Physiology and Evolution of Vision in Invertebrates. B: Invertebrate Visual Centers and Behavior I, Handbook of Sensory Physiology*, vol. VII/6B, H. Autrum, ed. Springer-Verlag, New York, pp. 281–469.
Weale, R. A. (1961). Limits of human vision. *Nature* (*London*) *191*:471–3.
Webb, N. G. (1972). X-ray diffraction from outer segments of visual cells in intact eyes of the frog. *Nature* (*London*) *235*:44–6.
Webb, N. G. (1977). Orientation of retinal rod photoreceptor membranes in the intact eye using X-ray diffraction. *Vision Res. 17*:625–31.
Wehner, R. (1976). Polarized-light navigation by insects. *Sci. Am. 235*(*1*): 106–15.
Wehner, R., G. D. Bernard, and E. Geiger (1975). Twisted and non-twisted rhabdoms and their significance for polarization detection in the bee. *J. Comp. Physiol. 104*:225–45.
Weinstein, G. W., R. R. Hobson, and J. E. Dowling (1967). Light and dark adaptation in the isolated rat retina. *Nature* (*London*) *215*:134–8.
Weller, M., N. Virmaux, and P. Mandel (1975). Light-stimulated phosphorylation of rhodopsin in the retina: the presence of a protein kinase that is specific for photobleached rhodopsin. *Proc. Natl. Acad. Sci. U.S.A. 72*:381–5.
Westheimer, G. (1965). Visual acuity. *Annu. Rev. Physiol. 16*:359–89.
Westheimer, G. (1979). The spatial sense of the eye. *Invest. Ophthalmol. Visual Sci. 18*:893–912.
Wheeler, G. L. and M. W. Bitensky (1977). A light-activated GTPase in vertebrate photoreceptors: regulation of light-activated cyclic GMP phosphodiesterase. *Proc. Natl. Acad. Sci. U.S.A. 74*:4238–42.
White, R. H. and E. Lord (1975). Diminution and enlargement of the mosquito rhabdom in light and darkness. *J. Gen. Physiol. 65*:583–98.
Williams, L. W. (1909). *The Anatomy of the Common Squid, Loligo peali, Leseuer*. Brill, Leiden, Holland.
Williams, T. P. (1968). Photolysis of metarhodopsin II: rates of production of P470 and rhodopsin. *Vision Res. 8*:1457–66.
Williams, T. P. (1974). Upper limits to the bleaching of rhodopsin by high intensity flashes. *Vision Res. 14*:603–7.

Wong, F. (1978). Nature of light-induced conductance changes in ventral photoreceptors of *Limulus*. *Nature (London)* *276*:76–9.

Woodruff, M. L. and M. D. Bownds (1979). Amplitude, kinetics and reversibility of a light-induced decrease in guanosine 3′,5′-cyclic monophosphate in frog photoreceptor membranes. *J. Gen. Physiol.* *73*:629–53.

Woodruff, M. L., D. Bownds, S. H. Green, J. L. Morrisey, and A. Shedlovsky (1977). Guanosine 3′,5′-cyclic monophosphate and the in vitro physiology of frog photoreceptor membranes. *J. Gen. Physiol.* *69*:667–79.

Wu, C. F., and W. L. Pak (1975). Quantal basis of photoreceptor spectral sensitivity of *Drosophila melanogaster*. *J. Gen. Physiol.* *66*:149–68.

Wu, C. F. and W. L. Pak (1978). Light-induced voltage noise in the photoreceptor of *Drosophila melanogaster*. *J. Gen. Physiol.* *71*:249–68.

Wu, C.-W. and L. Stryer (1972). Proximity relationships in rhodopsin. *Proc. Natl. Acad. Sci. U.S.A.* *69*:1104–8.

Yau, K. W., T. D. Lamb, and D. A. Baylor (1977). Light-induced fluctuations in membrane current of single toad rod outer segments. *Nature (London)* *269*:78–81.

Yau, K. W., P. A. McNaughton, and A. L. Hodgkin (1981). Effects of ions on the light-sensitive current in retinal rods. *Nature (London)* *292*: 502–5.

Yeandle, S. (1958). Evidence of quantized slow potentials in the eye of *Limulus*. *Am. J. Ophthalmol.* *46*:82–7.

Yee, R. and P. A. Liebman (1978). Light-activated phosphodiesterase of the rod outer segment. Kinetics and parameters of activation and deactivation. *J. Biol. Chem.* *253*:8902–9.

Yoshikami, S. and W. A. Hagins (1971). Light, calcium and the photocurrent of rods and cones. *Biophys. J.* *11*:47(abstr.)

Yoshikami, S. and W. A. Hagins (1972). Control of the Dark Current in Vertebrate Rods and Cones. In *Biochemistry and Physiology of Visual Pigments*, H. Langer, ed. Springer-Verlag, New York. pp. 245–55.

Yoshikami, S. and W. A. Hagins (1978). Calcium in excitation of vertebrate rods and cones: retinal efflux of calcium studied with dichlorophosphonazo III. *Ann. N.Y. Acad. Sci.* *307*:545–61.

Yoshikami, S. and G. N. Nöll (1978). Isolated retinas synthesize visual pigments from retinal congeners delivered by liposomes. *Science* *200*:1393–5.

Yoshikami, S. and G. N. Nöll (1979). The outer segment plasma membrane reveals the pigment epithelium to be the source of the 11-*cis* retinaldehyde in rods. *Biophys. J.* *25*(2, Pt. 2):314(abstr.).

Yoshikami, S., J. S. George, and W. A. Hagins (1980). Light-induced calcium fluxes from outer segment layer of vertebrate retinas. *Nature (London)* *286*:395–8.

Yoshizawa, T. (1972). The Behavior of Visual Pigments at Low Temperatures. In *Photochemistry of Vision, Handbook of Sensory Physiology*, vol. VII/1, H. J. A. Dartnall, ed. Springer-Verlag, New York, pp. 146–79.

Yoshizawa, T. and G. Wald (1963). Pre-lumirhodopsin and the bleaching of visual pigments. *Nature (London)* *197*:1279–86.

Young, R. W. (1970). Visual cells. *Sci. Am.* *223*:80–91.

Young, R. W. (1976). Visual cells and the concept of renewal. *Invest. Ophthalmol. 15*:700–25.

Young, R. W. (1977). The daily rhythm of shedding and degradation of cone outer segments in the lizard retina. *J. Ultrastruct. Res. 61*:172–85.

Young, R. W. and D. Bok (1969). Participation of the retinal pigment epithelium in the rod outer segment renewal process. *J. Cell. Biol. 42*:392–403.

Young, T. (1802). On the theory of light and colours. *Philos. Trans. R. Soc. London 92*:12–48.

Zonana, H. V. (1961). Eye structure of the squid retina. *Bull. Johns Hopkins Hosp. 109*:185–205.

Zorn, M. and S. Futterman (1971). Properties of rhodopsin dependent on associated phospholipid. *J. Biol. Chem. 246*:881–6.

INDEX

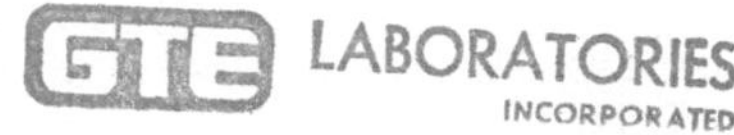

The letter "f" following a page number refers to the figure on that page.

CHARGED TO:

DATE	
7/15/83	[illegible]